The California Medical Marijuana Patients Book

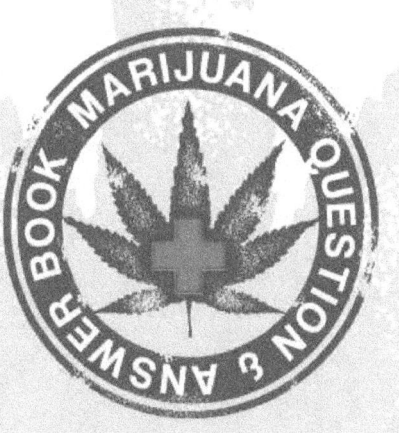

By
T. Oliver

THE CALIFORNIA MEDICAL MARIJUANA PATIENTS BOOK

For **free updates** of this book, or **free previews** of Oliver's next release visit us at:

www.mmpatientid.com

T. OLIVER

THE CALIFORNIA MEDICAL MARIJUANA PATIENTS BOOK
@2013 By T Oliver. All Rights Reserved

ISBN-13: 978-1493568949
ISBN-10: 1493568949

This Trade Paperback Original Is Published By
Four Twenty Press
Santa Rosa, CA 95403
www.fourtwentypress.com
info@fourtwentypress.com

THE CALIFORNIA MEDICAL MARIJUANA PATIENTS BOOK COPYRIGHT © 2013 BY FOUR TWENTY PRESS. ALL RIGHTS RESERVED. PRINTED IN THE UNITED STATES OF AMERICA. NO PART OF THIS BOOK MAY BE USED OR REPRODUCED IN ANY MANNER WHATSOEVER WITHOUT WRITTEN PERMISSION. FOR INFORMATION CONTACT info@fourtwentypress.com

THE CALIFORNIA MEDICAL MARIJUANA PATIENTS BOOK IS INTENDED FOR ADULTS, AGE 18 AND OVER. THIS BOOK IS SOLEY FOR INFORMATIONAL AND EDUCATIONAL PURPOSES AND IS NOT MEDICAL OR LEGAL ADVICE. PLEASE CONSULT WITH A MEDICAL PROFESSIONAL BEFORE BEGINNING ANY NEW TREATMENT PLAN.

FIRST EDITION

CREDITS
COVER AND INTERIOR DESIGN BY T. OLIVER

MEDICAL MARIJUANA PATIENTS BOOK IS A TRADEMARK OF FOUR TWENTY PRESS.
ALL RIGHTS RESERVED

ADVERTISING SPACE IS AVAILABLE FOR THIS BOOK
CONTACT US AT info@fourtwentypress.com

THE CALIFORNIA MEDICAL MARIJUANA PATIENTS BOOK

T. OLIVER

Table of Contents

INTRODUCTION ix

Notes About the Book xi

Dedication xiv

CHAPTER ONE 1
California Laws 1

CHAPTER TWO 5
Legal Q & A 5

CHAPTER THREE 31
Doctors Q & A 31

CHAPTER FOUR 43
Identification Cards Q & A 43

CHAPTER FIVE 67
Dispensaries, Collectives, and Clubs Q & A 67

CHAPTER SIX 83
Health Q & A 83

CHAPTER SEVEN 91
Marijuana Q & A 91

CHAPTER EIGHT 141
Growing Q & A 141

About the Author 150

THE CALIFORNIA MEDICAL MARIJUANA PATIENTS BOOK

T. OLIVER

INTRODUCTION

This project was born to give you instant answers. It's your one-stop resource.

When I first decided to seek a marijuana recommendation I searched for a resource to fast track me to the answers. I needed answers before I received my recommendation and I later realized I needed them even more after getting my recommendation. Even if you already have your card, this is a great resource. Through this process I found answers to questions I had always wondered about and learned an incredible amount of information; some answers even surprised me. This is information that every patient should know.

I found lots of books on the science of marijuana, growing it and even opening up collectives. There are a few books for patients; many go through every single possible use for marijuana and how marijuana helps it and I don't know about you but I don't need a book with 100 pages of reading on conditions that I don't have. I have a couple of those conditions so why should I buy a book when 50% of it doesn't even apply to me? I found other books for patients that were poorly written or they lacked the easy access to the answers I was seeking. I didn't want to read a 300-page book; I just wanted instant answers.

I have spent many hours researching answers to the most

THE CALIFORNIA MEDICAL MARIJUANA PATIENTS BOOK

important questions. I researched online, participated in message boards, spoke to people in the medical marijuana business and read about current news and legal cases surrounding medical marijuana in California.

This book is not meant as legal or medical advice; I am not a lawyer or a doctor and will not bore you with an abundance of legal and medical advice. I am a patient. I used to be a patient with questions but after much research and speaking to people in the industry I now have the answers and I want to share them with you.

When I first received my recommendation, I had not used marijuana in many years and I was lost. I was even a little nervous about going to a dispensary or club for the first time. Where do I find them? Are they all created equal? How do I find the better dispensaries? What makes a 'good' dispensary? What kinds of medications are available and in what form? Some information was easy to find while other things were extremely vague.

Learn how to get free medication and how to find the best deals. What's the difference between budder, wax or oil? Where do I find a doctor to get a recommendation? Is there a state card? Do I need an ID card or just a recommendation? Was my need for medical cannabis covered under Prop 215? Can I get a card as an out-of-state resident? Can this affect my job? How much can I possess legally? How much can I grow? Can I grow in my apartment or rental home? What are the laws pertaining to owning a gun while being a medical marijuana patient?

Use Amazon's Check Inside feature to read the beginning of

my book; I've included an index of questions in the front of the book so that you can see every topic I cover.

I want you to be happy with this book. If you have a question that wasn't answered by this book feel free to check my site and shoot me an email and I'll try my best to find the answer; I may even include your question and the answer in an updated version of this book (updates will be free for anyone who already bought the book).

www.mmpatientid.com

THE CALIFORNIA MEDICAL MARIJUANA PATIENTS BOOK

NOTES ABOUT THE BOOK

I will for the most part refer to an establishment that dispenses medical marijuana as a club rather than always saying a dispensary, cooperative, etc.

I provide links to good products, resources, etc. and I use bitly.com to provide them. I do this so that if the links don't work for you the links are short, easy to read links that you can type in and still use. This is also better because some of the original links are extremely long and I don't want to fill a book full of long links and junk you don't need. If a link is an obvious one (like leafly.com) then I will just use the short version of the original link.

TIPS! Calls out important tips.

T. OLIVER

DEDICATION

This is dedicated to my friends and family, I am nothing without you. To my wife, who has helped me make time for writing. Thank you for your love and support, you truly make me a better version of myself. To my best friend, who has supported me, and offered advice from her years of writing and publishing experience all while 'going to the store'.

CHAPTER ONE
California Laws

CA Health & Safety Code 11362.5 Prop 215

§11362.5. Use of marijuana for medical purposes.

(a) This section shall be known and may be cited as the Compassionate Use Act of 1996.

(b)(l) The people of the State of California hereby find and declare that the purposes of the Compassionate Use Act of 1996 are as follows:

(A) To ensure that seriously ill Californians have the right to obtain and use marijuana for medical purposes where that medical use is deemed appropriate and has been recommended by a physician who has determined that the person's health would benefit from the use of marijuana in the treatment of cancer, anorexia, AIDS, chronic pain, spasticity, glaucoma, arthritis, migraine, or any other illness for which marijuana provides relief.

(B) To ensure that patients and their primary caregivers who obtain and use marijuana for medical purposes upon the recommendation of a physician are not subject to criminal prosecution or sanction.

(C), To encourage the federal and state governments to implement a plan to provide for the safe and affordable distribution of marijuana to all patients in medical need of marijuana.

(2) Nothing in this section shall be construed to supersede legislation prohibiting persons from engaging in conduct that endangers others, nor to condone the diversion of marijuana for nonmedical purposes.

(c) Notwithstanding any other provision of law: no physician in this state shall be punished, or denied any right or privilege, for having recommended marijuana to a patient for medical purposes.

(d) Section 11357, relating to the possession of marijuana, and Section 11358, relating to the cultivation of marijuana, shall not apply to a patient, or to a patient's primary caregiver, who possesses or cultivates marijuana for the personal medical purposes of the patient upon the written or oral recommendation or approval of a physician.

(e) For the purposes of this section, "primary care-giver" means the individual designated by the person exempted under this section who has consistently assumed responsibility for the housing, health, or safety of that person. (Added by 1996 initiative Measure Prop 215 §1, eff.: 11/6/96.)

California Health & Safety Code Section 11357

11357. (a) Except as authorized by law, every person who possesses any concentrated cannabis shall be punished by imprisonment in the county jail for a period of not more than one year or by a fine of not more than five hundred dollars ($500), or by both such fine and imprisonment, or shall be punished by imprisonment in the state prison.

(b) Except as authorized by law, every person who possesses not more than 28.5 grams of marijuana, other than concentrated cannabis, is guilty of an infraction punishable by a fine of not more than one hundred dollars ($100).

(c) Except as authorized by law, every person who possesses more than 28.5 grams of marijuana, other than concentrated cannabis, shall be punished by imprisonment in the county jail for a period of not more than six months or by a fine of not more than five hundred dollars ($500), or by both such fine and imprisonment.

(d) Except as authorized by law, every person 18 years of age or over who possesses not more than 28.5 grams of marijuana, other than concentrated cannabis, upon the grounds of, or within, any school providing instruction in kindergarten or any of grades 1 through 12 during hours the school is open for classes or school-related programs is guilty of a misdemeanor and shall be punished by a fine of not more than five hundred dollars ($500), or by imprisonment in the county jail for a period of not more than 10 days, or both.

(e) Except as authorized by law, every person under the age of 18 who possesses not more than 28.5 grams of marijuana, other than concentrated cannabis, upon the grounds of, or within, any school providing instruction in kindergarten or any of grades 1 through 12 during hours the school is open for classes or school-related programs is guilty of a misdemeanor and shall be subject to the following dispositions:

   (1) A fine of not more than two hundred fifty dollars ($250), upon a finding that a first offense has been committed.

   (2) A fine of not more than five hundred dollars ($500), or commitment to a juvenile hall, ranch, camp, forestry camp, or secure juvenile home for a period of not more than 10 days, or both, upon a finding that a second or subsequent offense has been committed.

CHAPTER TWO
Legal Q & A

Q: What are Proposition 215 and Senate Bill 420?

A: Proposition 215 is also referred to as the Compassionate Use Act of 1996.[1] This California Ballot Proposition passed with 55.6% voting in favor of the proposition.

Commonly referred to as Prop 215, this proposition allows patients in California who get a valid doctor's recommendation to consume, possess, transport and grow medical marijuana. This was later expanded to include protections for dispensaries, clubs and other distribution entities.[2]

Proposition 215: "Qualified patients claiming protection under Proposition 215 may possess an amount of marijuana

---

[1] California Department of Public Health (May 17, 2011), <u>Medical Marijuana Program</u>, State of California, retrieved June 23, 2011

[2] "California Proposition 215 (1996) - Wikipedia, the Free Encyclopedia." Accessed September 6, 2013. http://en.wikipedia.org/wiki/Prop_215.

that is "reasonably related to [their] current medical needs." (People v. Trippet(1997) 56 Cal.App.4th 1532, 1549.)

"On January 1, 2004, Senate Bill 420, the Medical Marijuana Program Act (MMP), became law. (§§ 11362.7-11362.83.) The MMP, among other things, requires the California Department of Public Health (DPH) to establish and maintain a program for the voluntary registration of qualified medical marijuana patients and their primary caregivers through a statewide identification card system. Medical marijuana identification cards are intended to help law enforcement officers identify and verify that cardholders are able to cultivate, possess, and transport certain amounts of marijuana without being subject to arrest under specific conditions. (§§ 11362.71(e), 11362.78.)"[3]

Read the entire Proposition 215 Language at the beginning of this book.

Q: What rights do I have once I have a legal recommendation?

A: Per California law, once you have gotten a written doctor's recommendation you will have the right to legally possess, consume, use, transport and grow marijuana medicine. The state laws provide limits on how much

---

[3] "Guidelines081408.doc - N1601_medicalmarijuanaguidelines.pdf." Accessed September 6, 2013.
http://ag.ca.gov/cms_attachments/press/pdfs/n1601_medicalmarijuanaguidelines.pdf.

medicine you may possess but the limits may be higher in your city or county as local municipalities are allowed to impose higher limits than the states; they may not pass laws to reduce the amounts under that of the state limit.

Q: What is the penalty for possessing marijuana without a recommendation?

A: Under California law, possession of less than one (1) ounce of marijuana is an infraction, punishable by a fine of up to one hundred ($100) dollars. This no longer carries any sort of criminal record with the fine. It's like getting a parking ticket. It's not even included in crime statistics.

"If you are caught with more than one ounce you may face jail time. If you are convicted of a drug offense you may also face a one (1) year suspension of your driver's license."

Q: Does the federal government recognize state marijuana laws?

A: The federal government does not currently recognize state marijuana laws and the Justice Department released a memorandum stating:

"Marijuana remains an illegal drug under the Controlled Substances Act and that the federal prosecutors will continue to aggressively enforce this statute."

This means that while the state and local governments will not prosecute individuals who have a doctor's recommendation and stay within the legal growing limits, but the federal government may choose to prosecute. That being said, the feds have not typically gone after individual

THE CALIFORNIA MEDICAL MARIJUANA PATIENTS BOOK

patients and small time growers. They prefer to go after for-profit businesses, dispensaries, and large grow operations. The federal government has raided many dispensaries and cooperatives in the past, and during the raids they have obtained access to all of the patient records of cardholders and they have not used them to pursue users. The federal government seems to focus on the big producers; anyone who isn't following current California regulations or recommended limits is possibly at risk of the federal government taking notice of them.

If you are a patient and not a business, and are following your state laws, there is little to worry about when it comes to getting in trouble with the federal government by being a consumer or small cultivator of medical marijuana.

Growing over the state limits elevates your risk, but many people do it, and few have issues with federal law enforcement. There are county limits as well; check local limits on the California NORML website (http://bit.ly/15Cw65z). There is very minimal risk of federal law enforcement taking notice when growing at these county levels. The penalties for growing over 99 plants is extremely high, so you generally find many grow operations under this number.

If you happen to be one of the few individuals who do have a run in with federal law enforcement, do not say anything. Do not offer any information or answer any questions. There is a reason Miranda rights contain the following saying, "Anything you say can and will be used against you"; you should ask for your lawyer immediately. By asking for a lawyer you are giving out the least amount of information, and making a possible defense much easier than if you keep talking.

Q: What are the current federal penalties for marijuana?

A: Currently federal laws are pretty stiff, particularly in comparison to California laws.

A first offense possession in any amount can carry a penalty up to one (1) year in jail and a $1000 fine.[4]

Sale Penalties

Offense	Penalty	Incarceration	Fine
Less than 50 kg	Felony	5 years	$250,000
50 – 99 kg	Felony	20 years	$1,000,000
100 – 999 kg	Felony	55-40 years	$500,000
1000 kg or more	Felony	10 years to life	$1,000,000

Sale to a minor or within one thousand (1000) ft. of a school will double the penalty.

---

[4] "FEDERAL Laws & Penalties." Accessed September 29, 2013. http://norml.org/laws/item/federal-penalties-2.

THE CALIFORNIA MEDICAL MARIJUANA PATIENTS BOOK

Cultivation Penalties

Offense	Penalty	Incarceration	Fine
Less than 50 plants	Felony	5 years	$250,000
50 – 99 plants	Felony	20 years	$1,000,000
100 – 999 plants	Felony	5-40 years	$500,000
1000 or more	Felony	10 years to life	$1,000,000

Q: Can I possess or use cannabis on federal land?

A: Possessing or using marijuana on federally owned lands is one of the most common cases where you may see an individual being prosecuted at the federal level. Given that the federal government does not recognize state marijuana laws, it's advisable that you not take marijuana on to any federally owned property, including but not limited to park land, forests, court houses, federal buildings, etc.

Some travelers, campers and hikers have ended up in legal trouble with federal law enforcement by taking their medicine with them on vacation. You can get into hot water by even driving over federal land. If for some reason they were to find you in possession, you would likely be charged at the federal level, and they do not recognize doctor's recommendation from any state as a defense to these charges. The federal government will attempt to block you from mentioning or using your medical marijuana defense in court on the basis that it's illegal at the federal level. This means that if you went to court, there is a chance you will have no defense at all. Use common sense and avoid taking marijuana onto federal lands or in federal buildings.

T. OLIVER

Q: Does the federal government or local law enforcement have a list of ID holders?

A: As far as anyone knows, no, the federal government does not keep a list of ID holders. In fact, the state of California does not even keep a list of names of individuals who are given recommendations or IDs. The federal government is not interested in the individual consumers of cannabis but they do take an interest in dispensaries, large grow operations, and businesses that aren't paying taxes, etc.

Even local law enforcement does not have access to a complete list of patients because one does not exist. The state of California database only contains the ID number and a photo; no names, addresses or other information is stored there to protect patient privacy. If you are issued a card from a private organization or doctor's office, the state is not even notified you have received a medical marijuana card. Each county has ID numbers and photos of patients approved for medical cannabis. Law enforcement officers may call a phone number to verify your recommendation only when they have the ID number.

You should carry your patient ID and your recommendation on you at all times for the best protection against arrest.

Q: Can I use marijuana and operate a vehicle or boat?

A: You cannot operate a vehicle, boat or other motorized vehicle while under the influence of marijuana. If you are caught operating a motor vehicle while under the influence you are at risk of being arrested for a DUI, you will likely be placed under arrest.

THE CALIFORNIA MEDICAL MARIJUANA PATIENTS BOOK

Using marijuana and driving doubles your risk of getting into an accident.

You should avoid smoking or using marijuana in your car, even when parked. Do not use marijuana while the car is running or the keys are in the ignition or you can be charged with a DUI, even while parked.

Q: How will an officer know if I am under the influence of my marijuana?

A: Most officers will go by the appearance of your eyes, how you act, and smell, etc.

There is a new Breathalyzer that was developed recently that can detect the recent use of marijuana. With the trend in medical marijuana laws being passed, and even a couple of states fully legalizing it, it's likely that these will become commonplace in the next couple of years.

If they don't have a Breathalyzer, they can ask you to take a blood test; blood tests are the most reliable measure of current THC in the system. Refusing a test is generally used against you and used as an admission of guilt.

Usnews.com ran an article with information on the new Breathalyzer, check it out below:

http://bit.ly/19E3nSf

TIPS! Do's while transporting marijuana

- Do drive carefully, go the speed limit, wear your seatbelt and obey all the traffic laws

- Do leave your marijuana in the original bottles and packaging from the dispensary/club as these are usually marked as medical marijuana

- Do carry your recommendation and ID with you at all times

- Do try to blend in and avoid drawing attention to yourself

- Do try to carry less than the state limit of one (1) ounce; staying under this amount means you will only receive the equivalent of a $100 parking ticket with zero criminal charges

TIPS! Don'ts while transporting marijuana

- Don't use marijuana and drive under the influence

- Don't transport your marijuana while smelling like it

- Don't carry more marijuana on you than you need

- Don't carry any weapons with you

- Don't use your marijuana in the car, while the car is running or with the keys in the ignition

- Don't carry scales or anything that would make an officer believe that you may be trying to sell marijuana

- Don't transport or possess marijuana on federal land or in federal buildings

Q: What if I am stopped by law enforcement while carrying marijuana?

A: How you look, what kind of vehicle you drive and how you dress may cause you to be under more scrutiny. If you

THE CALIFORNIA MEDICAL MARIJUANA PATIENTS BOOK

are generally a target of police scrutiny, then you should think carefully about what you keep with you. I am a late 30's, geeky, and I drive a family car. I get little, to no, police scrutiny.

If you are pulled over while possessing marijuana, pull to the side of the road, turn off the radio and keep your hands visible while the officer approaches the vehicle. Treat the law enforcement officer with respect. Do not offer any information to the officer unless you are asked for it. Do not offer any information about your marijuana or your recommendation. Answer the officer's questions and have your paperwork in order and you will likely go through a routine traffic stop and be on your way in no time.

If you are not under the influence then you should have little to worry about it if you have your recommendation or ID on you.

Most officers in California will let you go with your marijuana as long as you have a recommendation. Marijuana is so common here in Northern California, that our local community officer assigned to our neighborhood watch group told residents that they rarely respond to calls regarding marijuana unless it's for excessive amounts, a minor is involved or it's considered a nuisance. A sheriff's deputy that I spoke to stated that they rarely see marijuana related arrests and that when they do it's usually for very large quantities of marijuana (illegal sales) or instances where the person arrested had other more serious drugs with them.

Understand that law enforcement officers are taught that

T. OLIVER

marijuana is bad and so you may run into some that flat out do not see marijuana as medicine and they will see you as a criminal. If you have over the one (1) ounce limit they may choose to still arrest you despite the law; though again in California this is becoming less common.

If you're paranoid about police interaction and possible arrest and you don't always carry your recommendation then I recommend carrying less than one (1) ounce of marijuana with you. Less than one (1) ounce of marijuana is a $100 infraction (much like a parking ticket). If you are carrying more than one (1) ounce and you do get pulled over and are detained or arrested do not offer any more information or say anything to the officer. Immediately ask for a lawyer and do not say anything further. It is never a good idea to speak to officers when being detained or arrested; seek legal counsel first and foremost.

You should be aware that the police may arrest and release you, but that does not mean you will be charged for a crime. The prosecutors ultimately decide what you can be charged with, and any possession cases where you were within your legal limits and possess a recommendation are likely to get thrown out.

If you were under the influence while operating a vehicle or boat then you will likely face a DUI (Driving Under the Influence) charge.

For the ultimate protection against unlawful arrest or confiscation of your medication you can get a state issued ID from your county of residence.

THE CALIFORNIA MEDICAL MARIJUANA PATIENTS BOOK

Use your head when transporting your medication and you are unlikely to have problems.

Q: What if an officer asks if they can search my car while I have marijuana with me?

A: Police must have reasonable suspicion before asking to search your car. You have the right to refuse the search but they will likely override you and still search the car. Law enforcement does not need a warrant to search a car as they would for a home search.

If the officer smells or sees anything that indicates a crime is being committed they can search your car. If you have marijuana, it is always best to decline a car search as charges may be thrown out later for unlawful search. If you don't have more than one (1) ounce of marijuana on you then you are facing an infraction similar to a parking fine. If you have a small amount and a valid recommendation then you will likely leave with your marijuana. Some officers may confiscate marijuana even with a recommendation; though this is becoming increasingly rare after the 2011 decriminalization of marijuana. The courts in California have ordered police departments to return confiscated marijuana and pay damages after ruling the operation was legal.

Your best defense against this is to avoid this situation altogether. Don't draw attention to yourself, don't speed, follow all the driving laws and be respectful of other drivers. Don't blast your music or act like an idiot.

T. OLIVER

Q: What are my rights when I have interactions with the police?

A: There are three levels of law enforcement interaction. You should be aware of these as they determine your rights and how you should react. Remember to always be polite. Do not escalate any situation with an officer; it will not end well for you. Most of these officers are great officers just trying to do their jobs. Don't make their jobs more difficult or they can make your life more difficult. Remember, the goal is to end the interaction without getting arrested.

Level 1 - Casual Conversation

During casual conversation the police are not required to have any evidence or legal justification to make contact with you. During this level of interaction the person the police are contacting is free to leave. They can ask you anything they want but you are not under obligation to answer their questions. Ask if you are free to go and if they say yes, leave. If you are not free to go, then the situation just turned into a Level 2 interaction; detention.

Level 2 - Detention

During a detention, the police can hold you for a brief amount of time while they investigate further. A traffic stop is a good example of a detention. You must stop and be questioned and you cannot leave.

An Orange County criminal defense lawyer on JaneDoe.com explains signs of detention as this "Orders to stay put, demands for identification, holding your license or property and not giving it back, handcuffs or sitting in the back of a patrol car are all classic signs of a detention."[5]

During a detention, you are required to give them your identification and tell them your name. You are not required to incriminate yourself. Do not offer information to the officers. If they ask if you have been using marijuana and you say yes, you have just incriminated yourself. The police do not have to warn you by telling you your Miranda rights you during detention, though they can use anything you say against you just as if you were under arrest. You should always ask to speak your legal counsel before answering any questions. This will force the police to either arrest you on the current evidence or allow you to speak to your lawyer. You do not want to assist them in gathering evidence against you. Should they choose to arrest you; you just went in to a level 3 interaction.

Level 3 - Arrest

If you are arrested on a marijuana charge, again, do not say anything. Ask for a lawyer and get professional legal advise before answering questions. Answering questions without a lawyer present will only make your defense more difficult later.

Most of our nations jails are cramped and it's a possibility that you will be arrested and released unless you happen to

---

[5] "Interacting with the Police | Orange County Criminal Defense Attorney - Law Office of Joe Dane." Accessed September 30, 2013. http://www.joedane.com/featured/interacting-with-the-police/.

be in a more remote area where they aren't burdened by overcrowded jails.

At a level 3 interaction, arrest, the police have either obtained a warrant for your arrest or they have developed what they feel is a case of probable cause. They can search you and your belongings once you are arrested. You can be detained until your first court date. Many people are arrested and released for non-violent crimes due to overcrowding of jails. You should not answer questions and you should ask for a lawyer.[6]

Q: What if the police take my marijuana?

A: If the police illegally seize any of your property, you have the right to sue in court for its return or if the property was damaged you may be able to sue for damages. This is becoming more commonplace and cases like these are likely to further reduce these types of incidents; particularly when they come at a cost to the departments who take part in unlawful raids.

Police in Vallejo, California were ordered to return over 60 pounds of dried marijuana to dispensaries that were raided without cause while operating within state guidelines and laws. It's very likely this department will end up paying the

---

[6] "Interacting with the Police | Orange County Criminal Defense Attorney - Law Office of Joe Dane." Accessed September 30, 2013. http://www.joedane.com/featured/interacting-with-the-police/.

dispensaries for their losses as well. [7]

Read more at this link: http://bit.ly/1bUNXMd

Q: Should I ever consent to a search of my home, my bag, my car or my person?

A: Every lawyer will tell you, you should never, ever consent to any search. The reason lawyers tell you this is not to stop the officer from performing the search (they likely will still conduct the search); rather it's so that if the search is later found illegal, any evidence they collected will likely be thrown out.

One lawyer stated he said he always advises clients to state, "I do not consent to this search" whenever anything is being searched.

It is always good to seek legal counsel before speaking to law enforcement.

Q: What do I do if law enforcement comes to my home?

A: Do not let the officer into your home unless they have a warrant. It's recommended that you step outside of your home and close the door behind you when speaking to law enforcement. Do not leave the door open, they may use this as way to get into your home by looking for a reason to

---

[7] "Police Forced To Return Over 60 Pounds Of Marijuana To California Dispensaries | The Weed Blog." Accessed September 30, 2013. http://www.theweedblog.com/police-forced-to-return-over-60-pounds-of-marijuana-to-california-dispensaries/.

enter.

If they have a warrant, check the date and address on the warrant to confirm it's valid.

If they do not have a warrant, do not let them into your home. If they insist and enter your home without a warrant make sure you state "I do not consent to this search". Call a lawyer as soon as possible and do not answer any questions.

Q: Should I carry my recommendation everywhere?

A: I have to admit that I will often carry my medicine (small amounts) without my recommendation. I always carry my doctor issued patient ID with me and it's rare for me to carry a large amount. I should preface this with the fact that I do not draw attention to myself, I don't play loud music and I obey all traffic laws. I'm a professional, live in a nice area, drive an ok car and I look like the geek that I am and so I do not seem to have a problem with law enforcement pulling me over on technicalities or through profiling.

If I were the younger, college aged me, driving my old beater; I would likely carry my recommendation everywhere. While most law enforcement officers are genuinely good people, some of them profile based on race, the kind of car you drive, how you look, etc. Decide what is right for you. If you attract law enforcement like a magnet, you should probably carry your recommendation with you at all times and limit what you carry with you.

Q: May I elect someone else to purchase or grow my medication?

A: You are allowed to elect a primary caregiver, but only if your situation demands it. The caregiver can't be someone who just deals with your medications; they must provide other care for the patient to be eligible in order to be elected as a caregiver.

MMP defines a primary caregiver as:

"Primary caregiver" means the individual, designated by a qualified patient or by a person with an identification card, who has consistently assumed responsibility for the housing, health, or safety of that patient or person"[8]

You must be at least 18 years of age to be a designated as a caregiver unless you are the parent of a minor who is eligible for a recommendation. Caregivers can be designated in nursing homes, hospice, and other short and long term care homes and facilities. Caregivers who are designated by more than one patient must reside in the same city and county as the patients. If your caregiver lives outside of the city or county where you, the patient, resides, then that caregiver may only have that one patient designate them as a caregiver.

---

[8] "SB 420 Senate Bill - CHAPTERED." Accessed September 6, 2013. http://www.leginfo.ca.gov/pub/03-04/bill/sen/sb_0401-0450/sb_420_bill_20031012_chaptered.html.

T. OLIVER

Q: My employer has a drug policy; can I be fired if they find out that I use marijuana with a recommendation?

A: Yes, unfortunately the laws in California still allow employers to fire employees who have valid recommendations for even the most serious conditions. If your employer drug tests randomly, you could consider talking to Human Resources before you get your card; though I honestly don't see that ending well for you. If you test positive for marijuana, they don't have to fire you, but they likely will do so given they have a policy already. If your employer does not have a testing policy then you probably do not have much to worry about.

Do not use marijuana while at work. Do not tell anyone at work that you have a medical marijuana recommendation or that you use marijuana. Keep this private. Trust the wrong person and you are putting your job at risk. Someone at work that seems trustworthy could even accidently let your secret slip so I highly recommend keeping it to yourself.

Eventually the federal government will be forced to remove marijuana from the Schedule 1 of the Controlled Substances Act; this list currently also includes heroin and LSD. Once this happens, I am hopeful that the Americans with Disabilities Act will be able to provide protection for patients.

I'm astounded that patients who are choosing marijuana as a medication, as opposed to using addictive pain killers, are being dismissed from their jobs for something that is a private, medical decision; particularly when someone can be an alcoholic (not a medical use!) and keep their job at

THE CALIFORNIA MEDICAL MARIJUANA PATIENTS BOOK

that same company.

Q: What if my employer asks me to take a drug test?

A: An employer may only require a drug test if they have a drug testing policy. If they do request a drug test, you have a few options. You can tell them up front that you have a recommendation and try to make your case and hope that they don't fire you, but it's likely to end in you losing your job.

If you can't afford to lose your job, your other option is pass the test by flushing out your system.

Most employers use urinalysis to test for drugs because it's the least expensive option. Flushing your system with tea, cranberry juice or water that contains diuretics can easily help pass urinalysis. If you decide to use this method, you should take vitamin B-2, vitamin B-12 or Vitamin C to add some color to your urine because flushing causes it to be clear. Some people have used Midol to reduce the metabolites in their bodies (which is what the test uses to detect THC).

Google 'How to pass a urine drug test' and you will find many methods that work.

When I was 20 years old, I had a decent job for someone my age and I liked it, but I was offered another job and I wasn't sure I wanted to change. The employer required that I take a urinalysis drug test as part of the pre-screening. I was a daily smoker of marijuana then and decided I would take the test after trying to flush out my system. I wasn't sure I even wanted the job so being young and dumb I figured why not see if I could beat a urinalysis without stopping smoking.

Back then, some company sold tea that claimed to flush out your system so that you would test clean. Little did I know that nearly any tea with diuretics would have worked. Essentially, I had to make up three quarts of tea and divide them up and then drink so much per hour before the test. For four hours before the test, I drank a lot of tea. I had to use the bathroom every 15-20 minutes during the flushing. I smoked marijuana just before going to take my test. I took Vitamin C to help give my urine a more natural color. I passed the test. I have to say that even I was surprised that I actually passed it when I smoked marijuana each day and never stopped. Flushing your system works.

Here is a link to the tea and instructions.

http://bit.ly/18KzmMp

Q: How long does marijuana stay in my system?

A: Marijuana can be detected in urine, saliva, blood and hair. How long it can be detected by these tests depends on the tests sensitivity and type of the test, how much you have used, how potent the medicine, frequency of use, your metabolism, and many other factors.

Typically consumers who only smoke or use once, are likely free of marijuana in just a few days and can take a urinalysis test and pass. Heavy, everyday users can expect to be clean of marijuana in 7-14 days with some users taking as long as 21 days with more sensitive tests.

THE CALIFORNIA MEDICAL MARIJUANA PATIENTS BOOK

The California NORML organization has a great guide on drug testing and times.

California NORML - http://bit.ly/GYn0K2

Q: Can I travel outside of the state with my recommendation?

A: Michigan, Arizona and Montana have reciprocity (meaning that state recognizes another states law) as part of their marijuana laws. Maine will allow you 30 days of reciprocity.

Rhode Island will accept recommendations from any state as long as it is for a serious medical condition.

Oregon will allow out of state patients to register with the Oregon Medical Marijuana Program. You are eligible to receive an Oregon ID card. You will need to obtain a recommendation from a licensed Oregon physician. This is only valid for purchasing medication in Oregon and those states with reciprocity.

Colorado and Washington have recently legalized marijuana and so you can transport your marijuana to these states as well.

Q: Can I transport marijuana on a plane?

A: This is another grey area. I have traveled with a small amount of indiscreet edibles (I favor caramels) and a pen vaporizer, e-cigarette looking device that vaporizes concentrates discretely. I've only done this when flying to states that have reciprocity laws that recognize other states

T. OLIVER

medical marijuana laws.

I have traveled with edibles to airports all over the country and to several foreign countries. It's a risk I take occasionally; I have a hard time being without my medication because I experience nausea nearly everyday.

Currently e-cigarette and handheld vaporizing devices are allowed to be checked or carried on to planes. I've carried my pen vaporizer on several domestic flights and I've never had a TSA agent ask me any questions about it. I disassemble it so it's several smaller pieces and put it in a little pouch with other things in my carry on. I expect these to come under more scrutiny in the future as people are stupid, and are likely to abuse being able to carry them on to the plane.

Be aware that you are taking a risk by traveling anywhere outside of California with your medicine, even when the state you are flying to has reciprocity laws in place. TSA agents may still confiscate your medicine and they may even contact local police.

Some airports are more marijuana friendly. San Francisco, Oakland, and Los Angeles are all known to be friendly regarding cannabis and are less likely to even bother asking about it.

Let me be clear, this is at your own risk and this does not mean that you are guaranteed to escape some delay, harassment or prosecution. Be polite, smile, answer their questions and hopefully you will be on your way.

THE CALIFORNIA MEDICAL MARIJUANA PATIENTS BOOK

Q: Can I use marijuana in public places?

A: For the most part, you can legally use your medication in any place that it isn't banned or posted as no smoking or is not one of the places listed in SB 420 11362.79 (see below).

You should choose your smoking areas carefully as it is still likely to attract attention in certain areas. You should never use marijuana in a running car or even while sitting in the drivers seat with the car off, as you can be charged with a DUI even while parked. You are allowed to use your medicine in your yard and on your property. Use common sense when medicating in public areas. Do not use it anywhere near any schools, student centers, youth centers, and recreation centers.

Be intelligent about where you medicate, regardless of the law, medicating in public may bring negative attention. You can smoke pot in public and few people will pay attention in some of larger or more eccentric cities in California.

I always try to be very discrete about using marijuana in public. I either utilize edibles or I use portable vaporizers so that people do not smell it. I rarely feel comfortable smoking marijuana anywhere outside of my home, with the occasional exception of an outdoor concert or even where there is an abundance of others smoking marijuana.

SB 420[9] defines where you may NOT use medical

---

[9] "SB 420 Senate Bill - CHAPTERED." Accessed September 6, 2013. http://www.leginfo.ca.gov/pub/03-04/bill/sen/sb_0401-0450/sb_420_bill_20031012_chaptered.html.

marijuana.

11362.79. Nothing in this article shall authorize a qualified patient or person with an identification card to engage in the smoking of medical marijuana under any of the following circumstances:

> (a) In any place where smoking is prohibited by law.
>
> (b) In or within 1,000 feet of the grounds of a school, recreation center, or youth center, unless the medical use occurs within a residence.
>
> (c) On a schoolbus.
>
> (d) While in a motor vehicle that is being operated.
>
> (e) While operating a boat.

Q: Are there more discrete ways to use marijuana in public?

A: Portable and pen type vaporizers are the most convenient and on-demand way that I have found medicate while on the go or in public. Edibles are an all day medication and I don't always need or want that much medication. I really like the Delta-9 O-Phos (bit.ly/19xRfjS) as my everyday portable, though there are many other vaporizers that work just as well or better.

Concentrates, when vaporized, generally have very little smell and attract much less attention than smoking or even vaporizing flowers. Some vaporizers put out so much vapor at one time that they still have a smell strong enough that you wouldn't use them in public.

THE CALIFORNIA MEDICAL MARIJUANA PATIENTS BOOK

Edibles are the ultimate in discrete medicating, though they are much stronger, last longer and are more difficult to get correct dosing. I use edibles when I have to travel to other countries. With edibles, I can take one dose and feel the positive effects of it for several hours. Because they are so discrete, I can carry them on the plane with me and take another dose if needed.

Q: Am I allowed to purchase a gun if I am issued a recommendation?

A: In 2001, the Bureau of Alcohol, Tobacco, Firearms and Explosives released an open letter to all federal firearms licensees stating that marijuana was still a Schedule I controlled substance and therefore gun rights are restricted. Never mind that gun violence is rarely, if ever, associated with the use of marijuana. Meanwhile, alcoholics with a history of violence are still allowed to purchase and own guns.

Federal law, 18 U.S.C. 922(d)(3), makes it illegal to sell a firearm or ammunition to any person that may be a user of a controlled substance.

When purchasing a gun they will ask if you use marijuana and if you answer yes, you will be unable to purchase a gun or ammunition. Lying while purchasing a gun or ammunition is perjury.

If you own guns, do not store your guns with your marijuana, as any crimes involving cultivation and firearms can result in extra charges and time being added to a sentence.

T. OLIVER

You may read the full letter from the ATF at the link below.

http://1.usa.gov/18cA60F

Q: Can I get a medical marijuana recommendation in California if I am a nonresident?

A: There is a lot of misconception with this subject, probably because of the rare doctor or club that will deal with nonresidents. You must be a resident to receive a state medical marijuana ID card that is issued by the County Department of Public Health offices. I have researched this and found that there are nonresident patients who have traveled here and have been issued a letter of recommendation by a California doctor. If they obtained an ID, it was not a state ID, but a patient ID issued by a doctor's office or another third party organization. Given that nonresident patients are not technically allowed to use our medical marijuana system, they may still have problems visiting clubs. Venice Beach is known as being an area that will give anyone a recommendation in less than five minutes, for nearly any reason, and many clubs in the area will sell to anyone with a recommendation.

Most doctors and clubs require that you be a California resident. Since some nonresidents have already obtained a California medical marijuana ID, then there are doctors and dispensaries willing to overlook residency. Now whether those people went to a shady doctor or they photoshopped a good fake lease or utility bill, I don't know.

If you are from out state and you manage to get a recommendation, you should be aware that this is only good

THE CALIFORNIA MEDICAL MARIJUANA PATIENTS BOOK

in California and those states with reciprocity laws. This will not be a legal defense if you are caught with marijuana in your home state. It is very possible that clubs may not sell to you despite your recommendation.

If you live here part time or even temporarily (college student, military, etc.), you can always establish residency here by getting a state issued ID card from the DMV or by bringing in a utility bill.

CHAPTER THREE
Doctors Q & A

Q: Can my doctor prescribe marijuana for my condition?

A: No, doctors may not prescribe any non-FDA approved medication or treatment. They can only recommend that you use marijuana to treat your condition. The FDA actually issued a statement in 2006 stating that marijuana should not be used as a medicine but that it should be studied further.

Patients must have a verbal or written recommendation; though I highly advise you get it in writing.

Q: Can my doctor provide me with medical marijuana?

A: Doctors/physicians are not allowed to provide you with medical marijuana or assist you in obtaining it.

Q: Which conditions can a physician write a recommendation for?

A: You can receive a recommendation for nearly any condition under the MMP guidelines because they allow a physician to recommend marijuana for the following list of conditions, as well as any chronic condition that limits the ability of a person to participate in one or more major life activities. California is one of the most lenient (other than Washington and Colorado where it's been completely legalized) when it comes to what conditions are eligible.

I find it to be an acceptable replacement for nearly any traditional pharmaceuticals with their long list of side effects. Even your over the counter painkillers have some serious side effects.

Marijuana is frequently recommended for the following conditions:

- Cancer
- Anorexia
- Chronic Pain
- Severe Anxiety
- Glaucoma
- Crohn's disease\Ulcerative Colitis
- Hepatitis C
- Arthritis
- Alzheimer's disease
- Lyme disease
- Muscle cramps/spasms
- Severe Nausea
- HIV/AIDS

- Epilepsy
- Spasticity
- Cachexia (Wasting Syndrome)
- Migraines
- Multiple Sclerosis
- Severe Stress

Remember, the physician is ultimately the one who decides whether your condition merits a recommendation, regardless of this list.

Q: Should I talk to my primary physician about medical marijuana?

A: You can talk to your primary physician; particularly if you have a serious disease. Large HMO, hospital and institution employed physicians are much more hesitant to recommend marijuana for treatment than physicians in smaller offices and those offices dedicated to marijuana recommendations. This seems to be the case, even when they are prescribing something with much more dangerous side affects, addictive qualities and something that is much more expensive; they will still deny patients access to medical cannabis.

Some caution should be used when deciding to talk to your primary physician as there have been reports of doctors at larger health institutions actually refusing to prescribe other medications to patients after finding out that they are using marijuana.

If your like me, this is particularly frustrating when that same doctor is willing to prescribe you Dilaudid, Vicodin, and OxyContin for your condition. Don't let this dissuade you. Our healthcare and insurance systems are setup for the benefit of the drug companies and corporations and they are still pushing dangerous, highly addictive prescription drugs for conditions that can be treated by much safer, natural medication like marijuana. I had been prescribed all three of the strong painkillers listed above along with a long list of other pills. My Kaiser Permanente doctor said she "was not able to write a recommendation" so I can only imagine that Kaiser does not look kindly on their doctors writing these letters. I predict that 15 years from now most of society will look back at the prohibition of marijuana and think it silly.

Should you decide to talk to your primary physician, be prepared for a rejection and even the possibility that they will try to dissuade you from continuing down this path. Remember, many doctors are ignorant to the benefits of marijuana and have been taught the same rhetoric that is pushed on law enforcement officers; marijuana is bad and has no medical use.

Q: Can a doctor be charged with a federal crime for recommending marijuana?

A: When Proposition 215 first passed, the federal government reacted by threatening physicians who recommend medical marijuana with possible criminal prosecution for aiding and abetting or conspiring with a patient to assist in the acquisition of marijuana. They also threatened revocation of the physicians DEA registration to prescribe any scheduled drugs, as well as threatening to excluding them from all Medicaid and Medicare programs.

A class action lawsuit was soon filed by a group of patients, doctors and non-profit organizations on the grounds that the federal pronouncements were vague and infringed on the rights of the physicians and patients. In April of 1997, United States District Judge Smith, issued a preliminary injunction to protect the doctors and patients rights. This essentially barred the federal government from penalizing any physicians for recommending medical marijuana.

Q: How can I find a physician who will give me a marijuana recommendation?

A: I recommend searching on Yelp for reviews after you find a local doctor. Look for doctors who specialize in medical marijuana recommendations if you don't want to deal with traditional doctors who likely aren't even allowed to recommend it.

You can search for a doctor who advertises that they recommend medical marijuana on the following sites:

CAL NORML - http://bit.ly/1awE9Cp

MarijuanaDoctors.com - http://bit.ly/17B6Nl4

MedicalMarijuana.com - http://bit.ly/17B6RkB

WeedMaps.com - http://bit.ly/1eku3IM

Q: How much does it cost to see a doctor and get a recommendation?

A: I've researched prices around the state and on average you will pay between $50-$150 to visit a medical marijuana doctor. Some places will charge less but then charge extra fees for things like a patient ID.

I went to Medicann and paid $125 for my first visit (ID included) and $99 for my annual follow-up visits.

If you're a disabled veteran you may be eligible for a discount so be sure to ask when making the appointment.

Q: Will my insurance pay for my evaluation or medicine?

A: Currently insurance companies will not cover the cost of medical marijuana or for the fees to visit a doctor for a recommendation.

Q: I know that marijuana helps my condition, but I have no medical records. Can I still get a recommendation?

A: Yes, you can still go and see a doctor and tell them about your condition, symptoms, etc. They will likely ask you if you have used marijuana and if it helped your condition. If you answer yes, you will likely get a recommendation, unless you go in with something really off the wall and even then, you'll probably still get it. Even if you have not tried it before or not had it in a long time you can get a recommendation for marijuana if it helps with that condition. Even if you have no prior documentation, you can go to a place like Medicann and get a recommendation. The doctor is able to assess and diagnose you his or herself; they can decide to give you a recommendation even without prior medical history.

You can get a recommendation for menstrual cramps, as should be the case. They are painful and reoccur once per month. Marijuana relieves the pain and the muscle spasms.

You don't need a medical history to get a recommendation.

Q: How do I get copies of my medical records?

A: If you're with a major provider who provides online services (such as Kaiser Permanente) you may be able to just login to an online account and print copies of any test results, medical records or prescriptions. This is how I obtained copies of my medical records.

If your doctor doesn't have online records, then you will need to make a request directly with your doctor's office. You do not have to tell the doctors office why you are you're requesting records. You should be clear what records you are seeking, which test results, which specialist records, and for what time period they should cover. You may also be able to have them just write a letter explaining your condition and the treatments that they have you on currently.

I took my medical records, as I have a disease that regularly qualifies for medical marijuana recommendations. In California, it's not necessarily required that you even have records.

Q: What should I bring to my appointment?

A: Bring a valid California driver's license or ID. If you do not have a valid state ID, you should contact the doctor's office and ask them what else you may bring instead. Some doctor's will accept a copy of a signed lease agreement for a residence in California, or a major utility bill in your name, etc.

THE CALIFORNIA MEDICAL MARIJUANA PATIENTS BOOK

If the doctor's office you're visiting includes a free patient ID then you should be prepared to have your photo taken.

You should bring any of your current medical records that might support your case to get a recommendation. If you don't have medical records, but you have prescriptions, you can bring in your bottles to show you have been prescribed medicines for a particular condition. This is not always necessary. I took my prescription bottles and medical records; I had no idea going into that it was so easy to get a recommendation in California.

I expect that some doctors are more stringent with what they will write out recommendations for but most of them in the business of writing recommendations are pretty lenient with them. If you're going to a recommendation mill down in Venice Beach then you will likely walk in an d walk out five minutes later with a recommendation.

Last, don't forget to bring your method of payment.

Q: What if I have multiple conditions that can be treated by marijuana?

A: I'm the lucky owner of more than one condition that would allow me to get medical marijuana. Like one isn't enough, it's so like me to excel at something lame like being ill. I digress.

I went to my first appointment with all of my information. When I filled out the pre-appointment paperwork it asked why I was seeking a recommendation and I listed out a few things. The doctor wrote the recommendation based on one of them and said to focus on the one condition over the other.

Q: What should I expect when visiting a marijuana doctor?

A: Most of the offices are small and have a reception area and waiting room just like any other doctor. You will need to fill out some paperwork when you arrive. You may pay your fees before or after depending on the office. Some offices have medical assistants that take your blood pressure, weigh you, etc.

Others just call you into an office with a desk and a doctor to discuss your condition. The appointments tend to be under 10 minutes.

Q: Do people get denied recommendations?

A: Yes, people do get denied, though it's extremely rare in California. I think it depends on where you're located, what office you go to, etc. In my research I came across a story about a guy who tried to get denied a card while living somewhere around Venice Beach and he actually went as far as telling the doctor he needed the recommendation because he had a fear of flying kites and that he flew kites for a living; he left with a prescription for anxiety.

The bottom line is, bring your records or just be prepared to tell them about your condition and how marijuana helps the condition and you are likely to walk out with a shiny new recommendation good for one year.

Q: How long is a recommendation valid?

A: Doctors may write recommendations for however long

they want but law enforcement generally only accept recommendations under a year old. I have heard that some doctor's will write a six-month recommendation; though I don't know anyone who has had that happen.

Q: Can any medical professional write a recommendation?

A: No, for a recommendation to be valid it must be written by a licensed California Medical Doctor, Osteopathic Physician, Osteopathic Physician Assistant, Physician Assistant, Naturopathic Physician, Psychiatrist, or an Advanced Registered Nurse Practitioner. These are the only medical professionals that can write a recommendation.

Q: What do I do with the recommendation paperwork I receive from my physician?

A: If you do not have a state issued medical marijuana ID, then carrying your recommendation is the next best thing. You should make a few copies and keep them in your car glove boxes, bag, etc. If you do not carry the original with you, you should keep it in a safe place. Many dispensaries/clubs require the original recommendation before they will let you become a member of their dispensary.

Q: Are all recommendations done on a yearly basis?

A: The majority of recommendations are for one year. Some patients will receive a shorter recommendation, such as six months. This is up to the discretion of the recommending physician so this may vary by office.

Q: What if my doctor issues me a short-term recommendation or doesn't issue one at all?

A: Luckily, in California, it's rare to be denied a medical marijuana card. If you happen to be one of the unlucky people who are denied, you have some options.

If you went to your primary physician, then don't worry too much, many physicians who work for larger health institutions will refuse to recommend medical marijuana.

If you didn't bring medical records or proof of your condition with you, then you should try to get the records and return to see the doctor again.

Your other option would be to find another doctor. I recommend that you go to a clinic that specializes in medical marijuana recommendations. They clearly do not have the problem of recommending this medicine as you will run into with doctors at large hospitals and institutions.

Q: Are there fees to renew my recommendation each year?

A: Most offices will charge the same or less for each renewal. Medicann charges slightly less for your subsequent recommendations.

Q: Do all doctors issue medical cannabis ID cards?

A: No, not all doctors' will issue patient ID cards. Some doctors will charge extra for an ID card while others will include them for free. Do some research and ask questions before you make an appointment so that you know what you are getting for the fees you will pay. Many of the chains

THE CALIFORNIA MEDICAL MARIJUANA PATIENTS BOOK

that open multiple locations will offer a free card as a way to attract patients. The larger chains are obviously more recognizable and therefore more likely to be accepted by law enforcement. Many of these offices even offer a free online or phone verification system so that dispensaries and law enforcement can use them to verify your ID is authentic and current.

Q: What should I consider before choosing a physician?

A: If you don't plan to get a state MMP ID then you may want to look for a physician that will issue you a patient ID. Once you find a physician or office, I recommend that you look up reviews on Yelp or Google. You will want to call and find out what the fees are for your visit and to schedule an appointment.

Q: Why did you choose the doctor's office that you go to?

A: I chose my doctor's office based on the name recognition, location, convenience and online reviews. Medicann is a large chain of offices in California, they issue a free ID with each recommendation, and offer an online and phone verification system.

T. OLIVER

THE CALIFORNIA MEDICAL MARIJUANA PATIENTS BOOK

CHAPTER FOUR
Identification Cards Q & A

County Programs and Hours

Here is a list of the current offices that issue the State of California MMIC ID. I've listed Websites where the counties have provided some information on the MMIC ID; many counties fail to publish this information on the internet. If there is no website listed, it's likely that that county does not publish MMIC ID information on their website.

A

Alameda County

Alameda County Public Health Department
1000 Broadway, Suite 310
Oakland, CA 94607
(510) 268-2977
Business Hours: By Appointment Only
Website URL: http://www.acphd.org/mmicp.aspx

Alpine County

Health and Human Services
75-B Diamond Valley Road
Markleeville, CA 96120

T. OLIVER

(530) 694-2146
Business Hours:
Mon, Wed, Fri 1pm – 4:30pm
By Appointment Only

Amador County

Amador County Public Health Department
10877 Conductor Blvd., Suite 400
Sutter Creek, CA 95685
(209) 223-6407
Business Hours:
Thursday, 1pm - 4pm

B

Butte County

Department of Public Health
202 Mira Loma Drive
Oroville, CA 95965
(530) 538-7700
Business Hours:
Thursday, 10am - 2pm
Website URL: http://www.buttecounty.net/da/215.htm

C

Calaveras County

Department of Public Health
700 Mountain Ranch Road, Suite C
San Andreas, CA 95249
(209) 754-6460

THE CALIFORNIA MEDICAL MARIJUANA PATIENTS BOOK

Business Hours: By Appointment Only

Colusa County

(Not yet accepting applications)

Contra Costa County

Department of Public Health
10 Douglas Drive, Suite 220
Martinez, CA 94553
(925) 313-1126
Business Hours: By Appointment Only
Website URL: http://cchealth.org/medical-marijuana/

D

Del Norte County

Department of Health & Social Services
880 Northcrest Drive
Crescent City, CA 95531
(707) 464-3191
Business Hours:
Monday - Friday, 8am - 5pm

E

El Dorado County

Department of Public Health
Emergency Medical Services Agency
415 Placerville Drive, Suite J
Placerville, CA 95667
(530) 621-6500

T. OLIVER

Business Hours: 8am - 5pm
By Appointment Only
Website URL: http://www.edcgov.us

F

Fresno County

Fresno County Health Department
1221 Fulton Mall, 1st Floor
Fresno, CA 93721
(559) 600-3434
By Appointment only
Tuesday 8:00 am - 12:00 pm
Thursday 12:30 pm - 4:30pm
Website URL: http://www.co.fresno.ca.us

G

Glenn County

Health Service Agency
240 N. Villa Ave
Willows, CA 95988
(530) 934-6588
Business Hours:By Appointment Only

H

Humboldt County

Department of Public Health
529 I Street
Eureka, CA 95501
(707) 445-6200

Business Hours:
Monday - Friday, 8am - 5pm

I

Imperial County

Department of Public Health
935 Broadway
El Centro, CA 92243
(760) 482-4438
Business Hours:
Monday - Friday, 9am-12pm; 1pm - 4pm

Inyo County

Health and Human Services
163 May Street
Bishop, CA 95314
(760) 872-4245
Business Hours:
Tuesday, 9am - 12pm
Thursday, 1pm - 4pm

K

Kern County

Department of Public Health
1800 Mount Vernon Avenue
Bakersfield, CA 93306
(661) 868-1220
Business Hours:
Monday - Friday, 8am - 5pm

Kings County

Department of Public Health - Vital Statistics
330 Campus Drive
Hanford, CA 93230
(559) 582-3211
Business Hours:
Monday-Friday, 8am - 4pm
Website URL: http://www.countyofkings.com

L

Lake County

Health Services Department
922 Bevins Court
Lakeport, CA 95453
(707) 263-1090
Business Hours:
Tuesday, 10am - 12pm
Thursday, 10am - 12pm

Lassen County

Lassen County Public Health
1445 Paul Bunyan Road
Susanville, CA 96130
(530) 251-8183
Business Hours:
Tuesday, 1pm – 4pm

THE CALIFORNIA MEDICAL MARIJUANA PATIENTS BOOK

Los Angeles County

Department of Public Health
241 N. Figueroa Street, Room 128
Los Angeles, CA 90012
(866) 621-2204
Business Hours:
Tuesday - Thursday, 8am - 12pm; 1pm - 4pm
Website URL: http://publichealth.lacounty.gov/mmip/

M

Madera County

County Public Health Department
14215 Road 28
Madera, CA 93638
(559) 675-7893
Business Hours:
Mondays, 8:30 am - 11:30 am

Marin County

Department of Health & Human Services
Office of Vital Records
10 North San Pedro Road, Room 1014
San Rafael, CA 94903
(415) 473-3288
Business Hours:
Monday - Friday, 9am - 12pm; 1pm - 4pm

T. OLIVER

Mariposa County

Mariposa County Health Department
5085 Bullion Street
Mariposa, CA 95338
(209) 966-3689
Business Hours:
Monday - Friday, 8am - 5pm
Thursday, by appointment only

Mendocino County

Department of Public Health
1120 South Dora Street
Ukiah, CA 95482
(707) 472-2784
Business Hours:
Tuesday, 2pm - 6pm
Thursday, by appointment only
Website URL: http://www.co.mendocino.ca.us

Merced County

Department of Public Health
260 East 15th Street
Merced, CA 95340
(209) 381-1015
Business Hours:
Los Banos: Tuesday, 1pm - 4pm
Merced: Wednesday, 9am - 4pm
Website URL: https://www.co.merced.ca.us

THE CALIFORNIA MEDICAL MARIJUANA PATIENTS BOOK

Modoc County

Department of Public Health
441 North Main Street
Alturas, CA 96101
(530) 233-6311
Business Hours:
Monday - Friday, 8:30am - 5pm
By Appointment Only

Mono County

Mono County Health Department
437 Old Mammoth Road, #Q
Mammoth Lakes, CA 93546
(760) 924-1830
Business Hours:
Monday - Friday, 9:00am - 5pm
By Appointment Only

Monterey County

Monterey County Health Department
1270 Natividad Road
Salinas, CA 93906
(831)755-5013

N

Napa County

Department of Public Health
2344 Old Sonoma Road, Building G
Napa, CA 94559

T. OLIVER

(707) 472-2784
Business Hours:
Thursday, 2pm-4pm
By Appointment Only

Nevada County

Department of Public Health
500 Crown Point Circle, Ste. 110
Grass Valley, CA 95945
(530) 265-1450
Business Hours:
Monday - Friday, 8am - 5pm
By Appointment Only

O

Orange County

Department of Health
1200 N. Main Street #100-A
Santa Ana, CA 92701
(714) 480-6712
Business Hours:
Monday - Friday, 8am - 12pm; 1pm - 4pm

P

Placer County

Community Health
11484 B Avenue
Auburn, CA 95603
(530) 889-7158

THE CALIFORNIA MEDICAL MARIJUANA PATIENTS BOOK

Business Hours:
Monday - Friday, 8am - 11:30am; 1pm - 4:30pm
By Appointment Only

Plumas County

Public Health Agency
270 County Hospital Road, Suite 111
Quincy, CA 95971
(530) 283-6330
Business Hours:
By Appointment Only

R

Riverside County

Department of Public Health
3900 Sherman Drive, Suite G
Riverside, CA 92503
(888) 358-7932
Business Hours:
Monday – Wednesday
7:30am to 12:00pm and 1:00pm to 3:30pm

Website URL: http://www.rivcommic.org/

S

Sacramento County

Department of Health and Human Services
7001 A East Parkway, Suite 650
Sacramento, CA 95823
(916) 875-5345

T. OLIVER

Wednesday, 9am - 4pm
Friday, 9am - 4pm
By Appointment Only
Website URL: http://www.dhhs.saccounty.net/

San Benito County

Department of Health & Human Services
1111 San Felipe Road, Suite 102
Hollister, CA 95023
(831) 636-4011
Business Hours:
1st & 3rd Tuesday of the month, 1:30pm - 4pm
Website URL: http://www.sanbenitoco.org

San Bernardino County

Department of Public Health
340 North Mountain View Avenue
San Bernardino, CA 92415
(800) 782-4264
Business Hours:
Monday - Friday, 9am - 4pm

By Appointment Only
Website URL: http://www.sbcounty.gov

San Diego County

Public Health Services
3851 Rosecrans Street, Suite 802
San Diego, CA 92110
(619) 692-5723
Business Hours:

THE CALIFORNIA MEDICAL MARIJUANA PATIENTS BOOK

Monday - Friday, 8am - 4pm
Website URL: http://www.sdcounty.ca.gov

San Francisco County

Department of Public Health
101 Grove Street, Room 105
San Francisco, CA 94102
(415) 206-5555
Business Hours:
Monday, Wednesday, Friday Only, 1pm - 4pm
Website URL: http://www.sfdph.org

San Joaquin County

Public Health Services
1601 E. Hazelton Avenue
Stockton, CA 95205
(209) 468-3404
Business Hours:
Monday - Friday, 8am - 5pm
By appointment only
Website URL: http://www.sjcphs.org

San Luis Obispo County

Department of Public Health
2191 Johnson Avenue
San Luis Obispo, CA 93401
(805) 781-4811
Business Hours:
Monday - Friday, 8am - 4pm
Website URL: http://www.slocounty.ca.gov

San Mateo County

Health System
Office of Vital Statistics
225 37th Avenue, Room 11
San Mateo, CA 94403
(650) 573-2395
Business Hours:
Monday - Wednesday, 8am - 5pm
Thursday, 8am - 4pm
Friday, 8am - 5pm
Website URL: http://smchealth.org

Santa Barbara County

Department of Public Health
345 Camino Del Remedio, Room 320
Santa Barbara, CA 93110
(805) 681-5150
Business Hours:
Monday - Friday, 9am - 11am; 1pm - 4pm
Website URL: http://www.countyofsb.org

Santa Clara County

Department of Public Health
976 Lenzen Avenue, Second Floor
San Jose, CA 95126
(408) 792-5065
Business Hours:
By Appointment Only
Website URL: http://www.sccgov.org

THE CALIFORNIA MEDICAL MARIJUANA PATIENTS BOOK

Santa Cruz County

Santa Cruz County Health Services Agency
Medical Marijuana Program
Santa Cruz, CA
(831) 454-3431
Call for appointment and directions
Business Hours:
Tuesday, 1pm - 4pm
Wednesday, 1pm - 4pm
Website URL: http://www.santacruzhealth.org

Shasta County

Alcohol & Drug Programs
2640 Breslauer Way
Redding, CA 96001
(530) 245-6426
Business Hours:
By Appointment Only
Website URL: http://www.co.shasta.ca.us

Sierra County

Department of Health
202 Front Street
Loyalton, CA 96118

(530) 993-6701
Business Hours:
By Appointment Only

T. OLIVER

Siskiyou County

County Public Health and Community Development
806 South Main Street
Yreka, CA 96097
(530) 841-2134
Business Hours:
By Appointment Only

Solano County

Department of Public Health
275 Beck Avenue, MS 5-185
Fairfield, CA 94533
(800) 273-6222
Business Hours:
Monday - Friday, 8am - 4pm
Website URL: http://www.solanocounty.com

Sonoma County

Department of Health Services
625 Fifth Street
Santa Rosa, CA 95404
(707) 565-4442
Business Hours:
Wednesday, 9am - 3pm
Thursday, 9am - 3pm
Website URL: http://www.sonoma-county.org/

Stanislaus County

Stanislaus County Health Services Agency, Public Health
820 Scenic Drive

Modesto, CA 95350
(209) 558-7191
Business Hours:
Thursday, 2pm - 4pm
By Appointment Only
Website URL: http://www.schsa.org

Sutter County

(Not yet accepting applications)

T

Tehama County
Health Services Agency
818 Main Street
Red Bluff, CA 96080
(530) 527-8491
Business Hours:
Monday - Friday, 8am - 5pm

Trinity County

Department of Health & Human Services
1 Industrial Parkway
Weaverville, CA 96093
(530) 623-8209
Business Hours:
By Appointment Only

Tulare County

Department of Public Health
1150 South K Street

T. OLIVER

Tulare, CA 93274
(559) 685-5710
Business Hours:
By Appointment Only
Website URL: http://bosagendas.co.tulare.ca.us

Tuolumne County

Department of Health
20111 Cedar Road N
Sonora, CA 95370
(209) 533-7401
Business Hours:
Monday - Friday, 8am - 5pm

V

Ventura County

Ventura County Public HealthA
2220 East Gonzales Road Suite 130
Oxnard, CA 93036
(805) 981-5301
Business Hours:
Monday - Friday, 9am - 4pm
By Appointment Only
Website URL: http://www.vchca.org

Y

Yolo County

Department of Health
137 North Cottonwood Street, Suite 2100

THE CALIFORNIA MEDICAL MARIJUANA PATIENTS BOOK

Woodland, CA 95695
(530) 666-8645
Business Hours:
Monday - Friday, 8am - 5pm

Yuba County

Yuba County Health and Human Services
5730 Packard Avenue 100
Marysville, CA 95901
(530) 749-6366
Business Hours:
Monday-Friday 8:30-11:00a.m. and 1:00-4:00p.m.
Website URL: www.co.yuba.ca.us

A to Z Listing of Medical Marijuana County Program Business Hours[10]

Q: Can I get an MMIC ID in any county?

A: Unfortunately, you may only apply for the state MMIC ID in the county of your residence.

Q: Can I get a recommendation from a doctor in any county?

A: Yes, you may get your recommendation in any California county, regardless of where you reside in California and where you will apply for a MMIC ID.

---

[10] "A to Z Listing of Medical Marijuana County Program Business Hours." Accessed September 7, 2013.
http://www.cdph.ca.gov/services/Pages/MMPCounties.aspx.

T. OLIVER

Q: What if my county doesn't have an MMIC ID program?

A: Even if your county does not have an MMIC ID program, you're still eligible to go to a doctor and get a recommendation and you can still use marijuana in that county. If you want an ID, then I recommend you seek out a medical office or doctor who will issue an ID with your recommendation.

You can also go to the Patient ID Center in Oakland, CA. IDs are available to all California residents at the Patient ID Center. For more information visit their website at http://www.patientidcenter.org/ The Patient ID Center is one of the most recognized organizations that issue ID's outside of the state MMIC IDs handled by the counties.

Q: Which card do you have?

A: I have a Medicann patient ID card. I don't generally have problems with being pulled over and I've never had an officer ask to search my car. My risk is fairly low, whereas your risk may be different from my own. If you attract the attention of the police, you should consider this and always carry your original recommendation and a medical marijuana ID. I have rarely carried even close to one (1) ounce of marijuana.

If you're petrified of possible police interaction and the consequences of having marijuana you should get the MMIC ID card. If you're unlikely to transport more than one (1) ounce of marijuana then you're probably ok (this is me) since they would likely either write me a citation and/or take my medicine.

THE CALIFORNIA MEDICAL MARIJUANA PATIENTS BOOK

Q: Will any patient ID card get me into a dispensary or club?

A: Some dispensaries, clubs, cooperatives and delivery services will only accept your original recommendation letter. Some will take a well-known patient ID as long as they can confirm the validity of the ID through a phone number or website.

Q: Can my employer find out if employees have been issued MMIC State IDs?

A: No, there is no way for an employer to search a database or list of names. This information is protected just as other health information is protected under HIPPA laws. The only way this can be released is with your signature or court order.

You are the best defense against your employer finding out. Don't go to work medicated, don't use marijuana at work, don't talk about it at work, and certainly don't ever tell anyone associated with you at work about it. Someone who seems friendly about it today, may use it against you later or even tell another person thinking they are trustworthy, so it's best to keep this medical decision private.

"All patient information is covered under the Health Insurance Portability and Accountability Act of 1996 (HIPAA) and cannot be released without the patient's signature or a court subpoena. The Medical Marijuana Application System does not contain any personal information such as name, address or social security number. It only contains the unique user ID number and when entered the only information provided is whether the card is valid or invalid."[11]

Q: Can I use my patient ID to get into dispensaries in other counties?

A: Recommendations and patient IDs are good in any county in California.

Q: Can I use my ID to get into dispensaries in other states?

A: Michigan, Arizona and Montana have reciprocity as part of their medical marijuana laws.

Rhode Island will accept recommendations from any state as long as it is for a serious medical condition.

Oregon will allow out of state patients to register with the Oregon Medical Marijuana Program. You are eligible to receive an Oregon ID card. You will need to obtain a recommendation from a licensed Oregon physician.

Q: Do I get a new ID card every year?

A: Yes, just like the recommendations, the IDs must be renewed each year, whether this is for the state issued IDs or the patient IDs issued by offices.

---

[11] "Medical Marijuana Program Frequently Asked Questions." Accessed September 7, 2013.
http://www.cdph.ca.gov/programs/MMP/Pages/MMP%20Top%203%20Questions.aspx.

THE CALIFORNIA MEDICAL MARIJUANA PATIENTS BOOK

Q: How much does a California MMIC ID cost?

A: The cost varies by county. You will need to contact you county for current fees. If you're on Medi-Cal you can request a 50% discount but you will be required to show proof of your Medi-Cal participation.

I've collected the current fees from those counties that publish them; if your county isn't listed, you will need to call the phone number for your county listed in the back of this book.

County Department of Public Health MMIC ID Fees as of fourth quarter 2013:

Alameda County - $103
Butte County - $111.15
Contra Costa County - $120
El Dorado County - $114
Fresno County - $107
Kings County - $225
Los Angeles County - $153
Madera County - $225
Marin County - $113
Mendocino County - $180
Merced County - $225
Napa County - $124
Nevada County - $170
Orange County - $150
Riverside County - $153
Sacramento County - $166
San Benito County - $137
San Bernardino County - $173

T. OLIVER

San Diego County - $166
San Francisco County - $113
San Joaquin County - $141
San Luis Obispo County - $131
San Mateo County - $98
Santa Barbara County - $108
Santa Clara County - $150
Santa Cruz County - $101
Shasta County - $106
Solano County - $200
Sonoma County - $160
Stanislaus County - $184
Tulare County - $100
Ventura County - $221
Yuba County -$126

Q: How long does it take to receive an ID?

A: If you submit all of your materials and fill out all of the forms correctly the county will review your request within (30) thirty days and will then issue the ID within 5 days. This means it will likely be a total of 35 days or less. If for some reason your application is incomplete this will delay your ID.

Medicann mailed me my ID within two weeks. Some offices will print them at the time of your appointment.

Q: How can a club or law enforcement verify my MMIC ID?

A: They can call a phone number or they can verify them on the California MMP website.

THE CALIFORNIA MEDICAL MARIJUANA PATIENTS BOOK

California MMP Website - http://bit.ly/1d6F1ny

Q: How can a club or law enforcement verify my marijuana ID issued by an organization or doctor?

A: This varies from place to place, but the best and only types of IDs I would consider getting will include a website and/or phone number that can be used for verification.

T. OLIVER

CHAPTER FIVE

Dispensaries, Collectives, and Clubs Q & A

Q: How do I find dispensaries, collectives, clubs and delivery services?

A: For listings of dispensaries, clubs, cooperatives and delivery services you can check the

- California Norml Directory - bit.ly/19yOdvH
- Leafly.com - bit.ly/16316CJ
- WeedMaps.com - bit.ly/1eku3IM
- CannabisSearch.com - bit.ly/1gdPtvL

Q: What is the difference between a dispensary, collective, or delivery service?

A: A dispensary is generally a for-profit business, which technically is an illegal business in California. A collective/co-operative/co-op is generally a not-for-profit cooperative of like-minded people who want to provide medicine for members and of members who want to buy medication from other patients/members. A delivery service is sometimes provided as an extra service by some clubs while other clubs may only offer delivery. Delivery only clubs can sometimes offer lower prices due to not having to pay for an expensive retail location.

I am a member of all three types of clubs. I will refer to ALL cooperatives/dispensaries/delivery services as clubs as a general term.

I was nervous about using a delivery only service at first, but after trying out a couple I have found one that I use regularly. I enjoy visiting clubs and being able to see all of their offerings, but I also am afraid that I may run into a co-worker or employee, and I prefer to keep my marijuana use private.

I have a delivery service that I use called Sebastopol Compassionate Care and I love the service and the product. I love SCC because the owner, Ken, grows and produces all of their medical marijuana and concentrates and so I get consistent, high-quality meds every time, and it's delivered to my home at my convenience. Ken happens to offer the best concentrates I've tried anywhere, hands down. If you live near Sebastopol, give Ken a call and mention my book. :)

Q: Are dispensaries, cooperatives or delivery services more or less expensive?

A: I thought that delivery services would be more money but they really are not more expensive. They all range in prices and pricing isn't determined by the type of club. You will find some clubs that price A+ top shelf strains at $40 per eighth (1/8) oz. and others that charge as much as $60 for an eighth (1/8) oz. You will find all three club types ranging from reasonable to over priced. Shop around and you will get an idea of prices in your area. Sebastopol Compassionate Care has some of the most reasonably priced, high-quality, medical marijuana, in this area.

Q: $45 per eighth (1/8) oz.? I can't afford those prices!

A: Not to worry. These are top shelf, indoor grown prices and in the Marin, Sonoma, Napa area; where prices are likely higher than other parts of the state. Nearly all of the clubs offer some outdoor grown varieties at very fair prices all while still managing to delivery high quality medicine. There is something for nearly everyone's budget. I avoid the clubs that price their top shelf eighth (1/8) ounces at higher than $45. I've tried the $60 an eighth (1/8) clubs and the marijuana is no better there than other good clubs. Keep in mind that you can also choose to grow your own medication at a fraction of the cost.

Q: Are all clubs equal? What makes a good club or a bad club?

A: No, clubs are not all equal. Just like any other business, you will find good and bad clubs, and some in-between. Some clubs have a more rigid, uptight and intimidating feel to them, while others are like going to visit a nice group of friends. If you don't get a good feeling on your first visit, try another club. The first club I visited was just ok, more of an in-between. The owner wasn't very friendly and the quality was so-so at best.

Look for clubs that have clean facilities. You will find small clubs with a limited but good variety of meds, medium-sized clubs with an excellent selection and then the giant commercialized clubs that have 50+ types of medication. I prefer the small to medium sized clubs because I like the fact that I become familiar with the staff and they remember who I am when I come in again.

Some clubs grow all of their own marijuana, while others buy from other growers and patients. Clubs that grow all of their own medication know where the marijuana is from, how it was grown, and can usually tell you exactly when they will have another harvest.

With the SCC delivery service that I use I know that I can expect quality. I've never gotten anything that wasn't as good as the previous crop. I really like this model of a club because I may buy an eighth (1/8) oz. of the Purple Kandy Kush strain and absolutely love it; if the club grows their own they will be able to tell me when they will have more of that strain back in stock. I can reasonably expect it to be just as good as the last eighth (1/8) oz. that I bought of that strain; particularly with indoor grows where the grower controls the conditions. It's becoming more and more difficult to find clubs that grow all their own product.

Many clubs buy from various growers. This is fine, particularly when they work with the same growers/suppliers and therefore get a steady supply of a product continually. This is the collective model. If they use regular growers then they likely will have more information about the product and how it was grown. Good collectives require you follow a certain set of standards to grow for them in order to keep up quality and ensure the safety of the medication.

These collectives are not to be confused with clubs that will buy nearly any medication, from multiple sources, and with little knowledge of the medicine. These clubs will sometimes carry a strain by a certain grower for a short time and then never carry it again. This is frustrating when you find a strain that works for you and then you get that again from the same club, only to find out that this harvest was by a different grower and is not the same quality as the last batch. I do not like this type of club, as I feel they don't have as much information about the medication and how it was grown and they typically just care about how cheap they can buy it and if it looks good.

I prefer clubs who grow their own medicine or use regular growers. I like a club that has a good selection of edibles, concentrates and flowers (buds).

I also like clubs that have private parking areas that are not directly off of a busy street. I have a professional job and would prefer not to be recognized going into or out of a club. If you are scared of being seen in a club (maybe you have employees, teenagers, or college-age children whose friends my recognize you), then think about using a delivery service.

Some clubs will keep the same small jar of buds on display for a long time. I don't like this, the buds lose their smell and get dry, and it's hard to tell the quality I will receive if I buy some. If a club does this, then ask to see what they will sell you to make sure it's not dry, only then can you properly judge the smell and look of what you're buying.

T. OLIVER

Q: How do clubs package their medical marijuana?

A: Some clubs pre-package their flower (bud) medicine and others will package it fresh in front of you. I prefer the later but will buy from some dispensaries that pre-package but it depends on how they package it.

I like certain packaging, such as the foil packs with clear fronts that are vacuum-sealed. In my opinion, this is the only way you can really get away with pre-packaged small amounts without them drying out. There is a club in Santa Rosa, CA that pre-packages their meds in orange/brown medicine bottles and the buds are nearly always dry. Fresh medicine should not be overly brittle, and it should have a fairly strong smell.

The regular medicine bottles are fine as long as they package it fresh, in front of you. If they are letting it sit in the bottles, I recommend inspecting the marijuana to see if it's dry and brittle.

Concentrates are nearly always pre-packaged in small glass bottles or small plastic screw-top cases. Typically you will find the thinner concentrates in the glass bottles and the thicker full melt concentrates in plastic.

Most edibles are packaged in plastic, foil, bags, etc.

Q: How do you find the best clubs?

A: Everyone will have a slightly different version of what they consider a perfect club. It's a personal thing and so we will each have personal reasons for choosing our favorites. I'm sure most of you are looking for good medication, good prices and a comfortable atmosphere.

If you have friends who have cards, you can ask them for referrals to their favorite clubs. When I first received my recommendation I actually didn't know a single person who either had a card or used marijuana so I searched online. Search the lists of clubs and dispensaries for reviews. Leafly.com and Weedmaps.com both offer lots of reviews on clubs. You can even find reviews on Yelp in California. This is a great way to start choosing one or two clubs to visit. Be sure to let the club know who referred you so that your friend will get a gift from the club for the referral. If you're nice, maybe your friend will medicate with you and share it after the visit!

Above all, the best method to find the best clubs is to visit them and find the one that suits you the best. Maybe you like concentrates, so you're likely to love a dispensary with a large and varied selection of quality concentrates.

Q: Can I go to clubs anywhere in the state?

A: You can visit any club in California, regardless of where you live or the county where you obtained your recommendation. As long as it's a valid recommendation, from a doctor licensed in California, it should get you access to all of the clubs.

Q: Are there any benefits to joining multiple clubs?

A: When I first started out I was nervous about trying out different clubs so I only went to a hand full of clubs nearby, once I found one I was comfortable with I just went to that one club. Then I moved across town and it was just too far to travel. This time I tried out a couple new clubs and delivery services, once I found one with high-quality marijuana, at reasonable prices, I just used that one service for a long time.

Then a close friend of mine got a recommendation. I introduced her to my two favorite clubs; really the only clubs I used. She later started researching clubs online and found a few she wanted to visit. She asked if I wanted to go with her and so we visited lots of new clubs over that year.

After this experience, I would say never limit yourself to a single club. They all offer so many different types and strengths of medications that it's good to get out there and see what is available at what price. This will help you choose your favorite clubs and find the most reasonably priced medication for your needs. The clubs I used to consider my favorites; I don't even go to them anymore because I've found other clubs that offer potent, quality medication at lower prices and with better employees and service.

Q: Is there an incentive to visiting a new club?

A: Yes! Clubs want new customers, they want you to try out their strains and check out the club; after all if you love their club and their marijuana offerings you will likely return. To get you to come as a first time customer, most clubs offer a first time visit gift. Sometimes this means a free pre-roll, some offer $10 worth of medication and some offer as much as a free 1/8 oz. of a top shelf! Whatever they offer, it's pretty awesome to get free medication. Sometimes you can find out what a particular club offers for first time patients by looking on the club website or you can try to check out weedmaps.com or leafly.com for reviews.

Try out as many clubs as you can. You will find better deals, meet lots of great new people and get free medication.

Q: Do I get anything for referring a friend to my club?

A: Yes, another great way to get free medication is to refer a friend who has a recommendation or as many friends as you can refer! Most clubs will generally offer both the new member and the referring friend the same gift. Some may offer something altogether different, but in my experience it tends to be the same as the new member gift.

I have referred several friends to several different clubs; when you think about that, it adds up really fast. I have gotten a decent amount of free medication over the years just from bringing in a friend who has their own recommendation and has never visited that club.

Q: Are there other ways to get free medication from clubs?

A: Some clubs will offer up another bonus gift if you leave them a review on leafly.com or Weedmaps.com. I've seen signs in some clubs that offer up a gift in exchange for a review. That being said, I'm not sure they will give you a free gift for a bad review so I'm not sure how good this system is for those that are looking for honest reviews. I've only gotten free medication twice for leaving reviews and this was only because I honestly liked the club and felt ok about leaving a great review and getting free marijuana for it.

T. OLIVER

I'm sure there are plenty of people who will leave a good review for any club, good or bad, just to get free medicine. The club may get a lot of people visiting their club to check it out but if the reviews are untrue, they won't return and return customers is key to the club being successful. If they are truly a good club, then customers will return. If they aren't as good as the reviews claim, then they will get a bunch of first time visitors collecting freebies.

TIPS! Are there any other ways to get free medication? (A very cool experience!)

April 20th is considered a sort of marijuana holiday. Think of it as the Black Friday of marijuana. 420 is a common slang term that means marijuana. If you're interested in the history of 420 and where the term originated, you can read how the term was coined in the next question.

I am sure that as marijuana is legalized and becomes more accepted in society this will become huge and commercialized and won't be nearly as cool. You should experience this 'holiday' in its infancy, before it's uber commercialized.

It was April 20th and my best friend and I had planned to go to San Francisco to attend a very large medical marijuana conference called HempCon; patients from all over the state were heading there. We heard that some vendors were giving out free medication at the event and that there would be great deals. Then we heard news that the lines were hours long and that it was so crowded you could barely get in, let alone go visit vendors and try to get something free before they ran out. My friend and I decided we weren't

THE CALIFORNIA MEDICAL MARIJUANA PATIENTS BOOK

interested in fighting large crowds for a free joint. We were both disappointed, but decided to skip HempCon and instead go to a couple of clubs we'd not been to before; we heard that some had good deals going on for 4/20.

We both started researching clubs that we wanted to visit and we came up with a list; we had no idea how cool it would end up being! We shared our experience with our friends who also have cards; none of them had ever heard of going to the clubs on April 20th.

Somehow, this turned into driving all over the county, visiting several clubs in one day; we dubbed it the 'dispensary crawl'. We visited several clubs and joined as new members, we even visited a few we already knew and loved. Because it was 4/20, nearly every club was giving out free gifts, bonuses with purchases, as well as the free gift to join the club. I took about $100 with me and I came back with a paper lunch bag full of pre-roll joints, kief, wax, medicated cookies, suckers, and cotton candy, as well as several kinds of flower/buds. I estimated that I brought home over $100 worth of free product, maybe more, and I saved another $100 because of the great deals and sales. Some clubs had some of the best deals I've ever seen. Top shelf indoor strains at one club were as little as $10 for 1/8 oz. Some places even served free food and drinks; a couple of them had full barbecues outside. A couple of the larger places had big events with extra vendors there. It was truly a unique day and it was a lot of fun to be able to see so many different clubs and their offerings. We've since told several of our friends who have cards about this and they can't wait until next year to experience it for themselves. If there is ever a day to hit up a bunch of clubs, this is the day.

Research the club websites, leafly.com or weedmaps.com and other sites that list dispensaries, clubs and delivery services. Many of the clubs will post their specials and even what the giveaways will be for that day. Make a list and prioritize based on which clubs you think are offering the best deals. You will not be disappointed with this day.

Q: Why is the number 420 associated with marijuana?

A: There have been all sorts of rumors floated regarding the origin of the term 420 (pronounced 'four twenty'). One rumor was that 420 was the police code for marijuana, another said it was the number of cannabinoids in marijuana; another rumor claimed it had something to do with the death of Bob Marley (though I scratch my head at that last one given he died in May, not April). None of these have anything to do with 420.

The term 420 was coined in the early 1970's in San Rafael, California. A group of about a dozen high school athletes, nicknamed, the Waldos, started the code word that eventually spread across the world. The name, "the Waldos", was started because the students would meet by the wall near the school.

The Waldos heard through friends that a U.S. Coast Guard service member had grown a crop near the Point Reyes Coast Guard station and he was no longer able to care for it. The group discussed it, and decided to go and try to locate the harvest for themselves; they agreed to meet outside at 4:20, just after practice.

THE CALIFORNIA MEDICAL MARIJUANA PATIENTS BOOK

Each week, they met at the wall at 4:20 PM and smoked marijuana before heading to Point Reyes to search for the hidden harvest.

From that point forward the group would refer to pot smoking as 420.

The group had some ties with the Grateful Dead community because a couple of their parents worked in the music industry. The Waldos would use and spread the term throughout San Francisco and the Northern California area. It spread throughout the US and eventually in the 1990's the term was noticed by *High Times Magazine*. High Times purchased the domain 420.com and began to use the term throughout the magazine and it's events.

Today, you will hear 420 used in various ways. You might find Craigslist ads for apartments or homes listed as '420 friendly'. It can mean everything from 'let's smoke pot' to 'someone is smoking pot'.

Q: Do you have any clubs you recommend?

A: I would like to give a free mention to my two favorite clubs.

Redwood Herbal Alliance of Santa Rosa, CA and Sebastopol Compassionate Care of Sebastopol, CA.

Both of these are excellent clubs with high quality and reasonably priced indoor and outdoor medications. I have never received anything except excellent medication and friendly service from them. *Redwood Herbal Alliance* is a club with retail location you can visit while *Sebastopol*

T. OLIVER

Compassionate Care is a delivery service.

Feel free to mention my name and my book if you go in; I can certainly always use some free medication for a referral and I love these places and want them to stay successful.

Q: Do clubs have sales like other stores?

A: Yes, many clubs do have sales. Look on review sites, the club websites, and leafly.com or weedmaps.com for deals and coupons. Some clubs have email lists that you can join and they will send out emails with special deals on a regular basis.

One club that I joined sends emails out at least twice a week with great deals that offer up things like a free eighth (1/8) ounce with any order, a free gram of wax or so on. Not bad when you can spend $35 and get $35 of medication as a bonus!

Q: What forms of payment do clubs take?

A: This depends on the club but most clubs take cash, debit cards, and credit cards.

Q: Are there any perks of going to the same club and becoming a regular?

A: Yes, but it depends on the club. I am a regular of a several clubs and they both will occasionally throw in freebies. I've gotten free edibles, even free samples of buds and concentrates. I appreciate the free samples the most, even when small. It gives me a chance to try out something new without investing money and it makes me feel appreciated for being a regular. Some clubs even offer frequent buyer programs where you buy so much from them or so many times, and they give you some free medication.

Q: Is there anything I should watch out for in the agreements I must sign to join a club?

A: So far I have not seen anything in an agreement that I felt I could not sign. Clubs that run as collectives will ask if they can include you in their grow counts. This means that another collective member counts you as one person they are growing marijuana for in the collective, thus increasing how much marijuana the collective may grow.

I've seen collectives ask patients to write down their medical conditions and I'm not fond of that practice; I choose not to answer it as I don't feel they need to know that information. The reason they usually say they ask is so that they can recommend strains that will treat your particular condition; though I've honestly not had very many use that to recommend something so I now choose to opt out of giving that information.

Q: Can I bring my friend, spouse, brother, mother, to the dispensary with me?

A: No, you cannot bring anyone in with you who doesn't have their own recommendation. Only patients and those people elected as a primary caregiver for a patient may go into a club. Most clubs will allow you to leave non-members in cars while you go inside but some of the more rigid clubs will not even allow non-members in the parking lot. I rarely go to these places; I find the later very off-putting as there are times I want to swing by a club for a quick pick up while I have a friend or relative with me.

Q: Can I elect my spouse, sister, etc. as a primary caregiver so they can go into clubs with me?

A: You can't just elect a primary caregiver so your friend or family member can go to clubs with you.

Remember that MMP defines a primary caregiver as:

"Primary caregiver" means the individual, designated by a qualified patient or by a person with an identification card, who has consistently assumed responsibility for the housing, health, or safety of that patient or person"[12]

If your friend or family member doesn't qualify as your primary caregiver under this definition then the only way for them to go to clubs with you is for them to get their own recommendation.

Q: Can I bring my caregiver or elect a caregiver to pick up my medicine for me?

A: Yes, if you do elect a caregiver, you can apply for a MMIC ID for that caregiver and they will be able to grow, purchase and transport your medication for you. The patient must apply for the caregiver.

---

[12] "SB 420 Senate Bill - CHAPTERED." Accessed September 6, 2013. http://www.leginfo.ca.gov/pub/03-04/bill/sen/sb_0401-0450/sb_420_bill_20031012_chaptered.html.

THE CALIFORNIA MEDICAL MARIJUANA PATIENTS BOOK

Q: What is the inside of a club like, what does it look like?

A: Most clubs have a reception area that is closed off from the store portion of the dispensary. You will generally walk up to an attendant to register or check in. Once they either register you as a member or check your ID to verify you as an existing patient they will let you go into the club. Some clubs have a limit on the number of customers that they let in at a time. This lets them focus on you as an individual patient so they can answer your questions and let you check out all of their offerings.

On your first visit, a good club will have an employee walk you through all of their offerings and specials.

Typically the clubs will have lots of glass display cases along with occasional refrigerated cases as well. Most of them put the fresh buds in glass jars. The jars usually are labeled with the strain name and whether it's an *indica, sativa* or hybrid (for more information on medicine types see The Medicine section). Some clubs will test their marijuana and list out THC and CBD percentages. Good clubs will have a good description of each strain and it's effects. They will usually let you smell the jars. Generally you cannot touch the medication; no one wants to buy what you've poked and prodded. I find that a description of the effects along with being able to see it up close and smell it is usually enough for me to make a decision.

Q: I've heard they can be scary, is this true?

A: Most clubs are warm and welcoming. Employees are usually friendly and professional and you are likely to have a good experience in most clubs. A very small number of clubs have less friendly staff and it can really put a damper on a visit. There is a really large, commercialized club here in Sonoma County that is a little intimidating; this same club won't let you leave people in your car in the parking lot. They usually have large, hulking guards and it's not the best atmosphere. It's not scary really, but it's not comfortable and welcoming either. There may be scary clubs but I have yet to really visit one that I would describe as scary.

Q: Does it cost to become a member of a club?

A: No, you will not likely see clubs charging membership fees. The only fees they should charge is the fees for the marijuana.

Q: Do I have to renew my membership with a club?

A: Yes, just like you renew your recommendation and patient ID you will have to renew your memberships with a club. Clubs will generally keep track of when your recommendation expires and they may ask you for verification of your new recommendation on a yearly basis. Some don't do a great job of keeping track of the expirations; this is really at their risk and not yours.

CHAPTER SIX

Health Q & A

Q: Is marijuana safe?

A: Marijuana is a very safe and natural medicine with a short list of possible negative side affects. We've all seen the really long list of side affects of our traditional pharmaceuticals; marijuana is generally going to be much safer than the average prescription.

This becomes particularly clear when you realize how many people die from taking over the counter brand name painkillers that nearly every American has in their home. There is no lethal dose of marijuana and no deaths have ever been attributed to marijuana.

"Regarding the relative safety of cannabis, former US DEA chief administrative law judge Judge Francis Young said:

"There is no record in the extensive medical literature describing a proven, documented cannabis-induced fatality....Despite [a] long history of use and the extraordinarily high numbers of social smokers, there are simply no credible medical reports to suggest that consuming marijuana has caused a single death. In practical terms, marijuana cannot induce a lethal response as a result of drug-related toxicity....Marijuana's therapeutic ratio is impossible to quantify because it is so high....Marijuana, in its natural form, is one of the safest therapeutically active substances known to man.""[13]

Marijuana has been shown to mildly decrease heart rates in some patients. Patients with heart issues should consult a doctor before using medical marijuana.

Q: Is cannabis bad for my health?

A: This book isn't going to go through all of the effects on your health; I'm not an expert or a doctor so it's important to do your own research as well but I wanted to cover some basics. There are so many contradicting studies currently that until we have more modern, legitimate studies on marijuana a lot of the long term effects are still unknown. Marijuana is less damaging that alcohol or cigarettes; for me that says a lot.

Like any food or medicine you put in your body, there are be negative and positive effects from regular use. How you consume or use medical marijuana greatly affects the possible negative side effects; I'll discuss the different methods in this section in further questions.

---

[13] "Medical Cannabis - Wikipedia, the Free Encyclopedia." Accessed September 14, 2013. http://en.wikipedia.org/wiki/Medical_cannabis#Safety_of_cannabis.

THE CALIFORNIA MEDICAL MARIJUANA PATIENTS BOOK

Because of prohibition of marijuana, studies in the U.S. on the effects of marijuana have been limited and unfortunately skewed. Many studies are put together specifically to support a certain standing so you may read one study saying marijuana causes x while another study says it prevents x.

Long time smokers can suffer from lung diseases like chronic bronchitis, emphysema and COPD. The biggest issue with marijuana is smoking it. While smoking marijuana is not nearly as bad as smoking cigarettes, you are still inhaling smoke with lots of toxins in it and holding it in your lungs. The longer you hold it, the more toxins stay in your lungs. If you're concerned about this then you should consider vaporizing or using edibles instead.

I loved smoking marijuana but switched to vaporizing after my mother was diagnosed with COPD. She quit smoking over 25 years before being diagnosed and it made me realize I needed to stop now or risk my health.

Q: Does smoking or vaporizing marijuana cause cancer?

A: Several studies that our government has sponsored (to support prohibition) to prove marijuana use causes cancer have shown marijuana actually fights and even helps to prevent cancer. Oops!

I picked up a printout called 'Top 10 Cannabis Studies the Government Wished it Had Never Funded' and I found it online. If you're interested, you can read it here:

http://bit.ly/1c7KSJR

Marijuana (when smoked) contains about 70% of the same

carcinogens as cigarettes. Studies have even shown that tobacco smokers who also smoke marijuana are less likely to develop lung cancer than those people who only smoke tobacco. Scientists think that this has something to do with the THC in the marijuana.

Marijuana has been shown to fight and control tumor growth in breast, skin, colon, lung and other types of cancers.

Vaporizing marijuana will remove all of those nasty carcinogens so if you're worried about damage to your lungs or cancer, vaporize. It's a much healthier way to use marijuana and it eliminates tars and most of the carcinogens.

"Cellular studies and even some studies in animal models suggest that THC has antitumor properties, either by encouraging the death of genetically damaged cells that can become cancerous or by restricting the development of the blood supply that feeds tumors, Tashkin tells WebMD. Several studies world-wide have show that even long-term, heavy smoking of marijuana does is not associated with higher risks of lung, colon, cervix, breast, prostate and other tobacco related cancers."

[14]Here's what 10 Facts About Marijuana on DrugPolicy.org says about cancer studies.

---

[14] "Pot Smoking Not Linked to Lung Cancer." Accessed September 15, 2013. http://www.webmd.com/lung-cancer/news/20060523/pot-smoking-not-linked-to-lung-cancer?page=2.

A more recent (2009) population-based case-control study found that moderate marijuana smoking over a 20 year period was associated with reduced risk of head and neck cancer (See Liang et al). And a 5-year-long population-based case control study found even long-term heavy marijuana smoking was not associated with lung cancer or UAT (upper aerodigestive tract) cancers.[15]

One study actually found it reduced head and neck cancers.[16]

Q: Has anyone ever died from a marijuana overdose?

A: Science has proven time and time again that it is impossible for a human to consume or use enough THC to cause a fatality. There has not been a single death related to overdosing on marijuana. You can certainly consume (edibles) enough that you will be unhappy and uncomfortable for up to several hours. Even over-the-counter painkillers cause deaths every year.

Q: Is marijuana addictive?

A: Most people probably don't realize that marijuana is less addictive than caffeine.

---

[15] "10 Facts About Marijuana | Marijuana Policy and Effects | Drug Policy Alliance." Accessed September 15, 2013. http://www.drugpolicy.org/drug-facts/10-facts-about-marijuana.

[16] "A Population-based Case-control Stud... [Cancer Prev Res (Phila). 2009] - PubMed - NCBI." Accessed September 15, 2013. http://www.ncbi.nlm.nih.gov/pubmed/19638490.

"Dr. Jack E. Henningfield of NIDA ranked the relative addictiveness of 6 substances (cannabis, caffeine, cocaine, alcohol, heroin and nicotine). Cannabis ranked least addictive, with caffeine the second least addictive and nicotine the most addictive."[17]

Caffeine is much more addictive than marijuana; I even found kicking caffeine to be much more difficult to stop because of the two weeks of horrible headaches I experienced when I gave up coffee. When used on a daily basis for a long period of time you will develop a mild addiction to it.

If you're a heavy user of marijuana and you stop suddenly you *may* experience sleeplessness, headaches and even irritability, though this is actually quite rare.   These symptoms should disappear within a week. I have personally stopped several times and never experienced any side effects, though when I stopped drinking caffeine I had horrible headaches for nearly two weeks.

Q: What about health effects on adolescents using habitually?

A: Regular use of marijuana before the brain is fully developed has been linked to depression, mental disorders, anxiety and at times even psychosis. Not many people realize that person's brain is not actually fully developed until the age of 24. Further studies are needed before we

---

[17] "Cannabis (drug) - Wikipedia, the Free Encyclopedia." Accessed September 14, 2013. http://en.wikipedia.org/wiki/Cannabis_(drug).

will know all of the effects on the young brain.

Q: I don't want to smoke, what are my other options?

A: I highly recommend purchasing one or more vaporizers. I have several and I almost never smoke anymore. I smoked my medication previously. I thought I would never stop smoking it even if I liked vaping it too. Now that I have a few different vaporizers for different situations and locations, I nearly always vape. I still indulge in the occasional joint with friends but after vaporizing for a while, smoking seems harsh and tastes bad to me.

You also can try edibles, tinctures, topicals and capsules.

Q: Are edibles a healthy option for medicating?

A: Edibles are an excellent way of medication while not inhaling something into your lungs. Edibles are probably the safest method of medical marijuana delivery to your system in terms of not exposing yourself to carcinogens and not damaging your lungs. As discussed in The Chapter Seven - Marijuana Section, proper dosing with edibles is the tricky part.

Q: Is it better to smoke, vaporize or eat medical marijuana for my condition?

A: Everyone is different; experiment with the different methods of consuming marijuana. Just as a doctor may prescribe you one allergy medication and then switch you to another when that one didn't work for you; you will want to try different methods and strains to see what you like.

T. OLIVER

I find that vaporizing and edibles are all I need and I feel they are the safest forms for me while being more discrete. I have stomach and intestinal issues and edibles seem to offer me really great relief when I'm severely ill. This is likely because edibles are delivering a larger and stronger dose.

THE CALIFORNIA MEDICAL MARIJUANA PATIENTS BOOK

CHAPTER SEVEN
Marijuana Q & A

Q: Where do I get marijuana once I have my recommendation?

A: You can buy marijuana at one of hundreds of the various dispensaries, clubs, cooperatives and delivery services around the state. You may also grow your own medicine or elect to have another person, caregiver, or collective to grow the medicine for you.

For more information on the clubs see the Dispensary section.

For listings of dispensaries, clubs, cooperatives and delivery services you can check the California Norml Directory (bit.ly/19yOdvH), leafly.com, WeedMaps.com, and CannabisSearch.com.

Many of these services also offer free smartphone applications.

Q: What measurements is marijuana sold in?

A: Marijuana is sold by the gram, ounce or pound.

Most clubs will post prices for a gram, an eighth (1/8) ounce (3.5 grams), quarter (1/4) ounce, half (1/2) ounce and one (1) ounce amounts. I will frequently purchase one (1) gram of a strain to try it out before investing more money in it.

Some clubs may not sell grams (most do) while others may offer an off-the-menu option of buying a gram; particularly if you're a regular customer. If you want to try out a particular strain and your club or delivery service doesn't post prices for a gram, just ask, most will be willing to sell you a smaller amount so you can try it out.

Q: How much medical marijuana can I possess if I have a recommendation?

A: MMP Qualified patients and primary caregivers who possess a state-issued identification card may possess 8 oz. of dried marijuana, and may maintain no more than 6 mature or 12 immature plants per qualified patient. (§ 11362.77(a).) But, if "a qualified patient or primary caregiver has a doctor's recommendation that this quantity does not meet the qualified patient's medical needs, the qualified patient or primary caregiver may possess an amount of marijuana consistent with the patient's needs." (§ 11362.77(b).) Only the dried mature processed flowers or buds of the female *Cannabis* plant should be considered when determining allowable quantities of medical marijuana for purposes of the MMP. (§ 11362.77(d).)[18]

---

[18] On May 22, 2008, California's Second District Court of Appeal

THE CALIFORNIA MEDICAL MARIJUANA PATIENTS BOOK

Counties and cities may adopt regulations that allow patients to exceed the guidelines of MMP; to protect patient rights local governments may not set the limits at a lower level. Staying within the MMP guidelines is highly recommended, as this will assure you are always within the MMP standards. Keep these limits in mind whenever you are transporting marijuana, particularly if you are traveling outside of your county, where the limits may differ from your own county.

Q: How should I store marijuana?

A: It is good to store plant material in airtight containers or high quality plastic bags. You want to store your marijuana out of the light, as you don't want it to dry out and get brittle. There are companies that sell airtight containers for pot but you can buy similar containers that are made for food. Canning jars are an excellent way to store marijuana and keep it fresh. If it does get brittle you can put an orange rind in the bag for a couple of hours and then remove it. Do not leave it in there very long or you will cause your

---

severed Health & Safety Code § 11362.77 from the MMP on the ground that the statute's possession guidelines were an unconstitutional amendment of Proposition 215, which does not quantify the marijuana a patient may possess. (See People v. Kelly

(2008) 163 Cal.App.4th 124, 77 Cal.Rptr.3

d 390.) The Third District Court of Appeal recently reached a similar conclusion in People v. Phomphakdy (July 31, 2008) --- Cal.Rptr.3d ---, 2008 WL 2931369. The California Supreme Court has granted review in Kelly and the Attorney General intends to seek review in Phomphakdy.

marijuana to get too moist and cause mold growth.

Cheap, thin baggies do not work well. Avoid the open sandwich bags and opt from something thicker and sealable. Many clubs and patients will use one of the many food-sealing systems that seal the pot in an airtight bag. Freezing is not recommended, but refrigeration while in an airtight container is a great way to keep marijuana fresh.

For those looking for superior storage methods, look at humidors. Humidors will store your marijuana at the right temperature and humidity; keeping it fresh for a much longer period of time.

Some people freeze marijuana but this can cause the trichomes to become brittle and fall off. If you do store your pot this way, you should not handle it while it's frozen, as you will lose more of the THC rich trichomes while prepping. Remove it from the freezer and put it in a refrigerator, and let it thaw in there. Moving the marijuana to the refrigerator keeps moisture from forming on the marijuana during the thawing process.

When I had a larger amount that would last me a long time, I used a *FoodSaver* to seal up portions of the plant material and remove most of the air. I put some in the freezer and some in the refrigerator. I stored it like this for several months and the quality and taste seemed to stay consistent. I could not personally tell the difference between the marijuana that I had frozen and the stuff I had just refrigerated. I would love to see the results of THC testing of some marijuana when it is first harvested, and then again after storage in a refrigerator as well as after being frozen.

THE CALIFORNIA MEDICAL MARIJUANA PATIENTS BOOK

As marijuana is decriminalized and even legalized throughout the country we will likely see more studies being done.

Optimal storage for pot is between 41-68F degrees and below 60% humidity.

CAUTION: Be careful with edibles and all marijuana products when you have children or pets in the house. Store them in a freezer, up high, or in a locked container or area, where children and/or pets cannot reach. This goes for all of your marijuana, but edibles can be particularly dangerous to leave out because they are strong and usually come with several doses. Keep in mind that when they are homemade and therefore not labeled, even an adult can accidentally ingest your medicine, so clearly label it and store it in a safe place.

Dogs and cats have been known to eat marijuana out of ashtrays, so don't be lax in leaving even this leftover material around or you could end up with a really ill pet. Marijuana is poisonous to animals, when they are exposed to it by eating it or people being stupid and blowing smoke in their faces, it is not a good experience for them or for their owners. They will likely have explosive diarrhea, may urinate all over and their heads will bob. This will cause the animal a lot of anxiety, as they do not understand why they feel this way. Do not expose your animals and do not let them eat edibles. If your animal is exposed you should take them to an emergency vet immediately, most pets will require hydration via IV and the vet may induce vomiting. Cats seem to have stronger and longer negative effects from marijuana, though it's less common for cats to eat marijuana products than dogs since dogs seem to eat just about anything.

Q: How does it feel to use marijuana?

A: Everyone is different and your experience will be affected by your mood, the type of medicine you use, how you use it, how you feel about the people around you, and more. While it's considered a mildly hallucinogenic drug not to worry, you won't actually hallucinate as people do on other hallucinogenic drugs. Until you are used to the effects you will probably want to do this where you feel safe and are surrounded by people you trust. Some users report not feeling anything the first time or even the first few times using marijuana.

Marijuana experiences are full of contradictory effects. One strain may reduce anxiety in one person while increasing it in another; too much can trigger some anxiety.

When smoked or vaporized you will feel the effects nearly immediately, though the full effect may take 15-30 minutes; after this point it will likely last for 2-5 hours. Smoking or vaporizing when first starting to try marijuana is probably best as the dose is easy to regulate because you feel the effects right away.

You will likely experience a sense of euphoria along with feelings of general well-being, relaxation and stress reduction. You may feel more creative with some abstract philosophical thinking. Colors may seem brighter and more beautiful. It may make you feel energized while another strain may make you feel sleepy. You may feel introspective or may find yourself having long conversations about nothing with a friend or family member. Because of it's often introspective effects it can sometimes give you a new perspective on a problem or situation. Certain strains can cause the fits of laughter you see depicted in films (there's nothing like a long hearty laughing fit to make you feel better).

Marijuana is often considered an experience enhancer. It can make a movie funnier or a trip to the store may feel like a mini-adventure. Playing games, being creative, listening to music or simply sitting outdoors on a beautiful day can be enhanced by marijuana. I don't recommend going out while under the effects until you have tried it a couple of times and you are comfortable with it.

You may experience some loss of motor coordination, dry mouth, dry and/or bloodshot eyes, mild increase in heart rate, problems with memory or difficulty problem solving or thinking clearly. You may be energized (*sativa*) or tired (*indica*). Many people get the "munchies" from marijuana while some others experience a loss of appetite.

Some people enjoy social interaction while under the effects of marijuana while others become quiet and self-conscious.

Q: What are the possible long-term negative effects of marijuana?

A: Some studies list a side effect of the short-term memory loss in long-term, heavy users. Users who smoke also run the risk of respiratory diseases such as emphysema.

Q: What kinds of marijuana are available?

A: Marijuana is not what it was 20 years ago; it's not even what it was 5 years ago. With so many states legalizing medical marijuana and even decriminalizing it altogether, growers, clubs and other marijuana companies are looking for new and inventive ways to deliver the positive effects of marijuana in entirely new ways.

Marijuana is either a *sativa* or an *indica* strain while others are hybrids of the two types. The effects of the types are different so you will want to find the type that works best for your condition. Read further for more on the strain types.

You can get medical marijuana in many forms and new strains and forms are being created all of the time. The most common form is just the buds (frequently referred to as flowers or plant material) of the female plant. You will also find kief, hash, concentrates (also called full melts), edibles (baked goods, candies, cannabis butter, capsules and other ingestibles), drinks, tinctures, topicals, pre-rolls and more.

I will go over all of these options later in this section, so read ahead!

Q: What are cannabinoids?

A: Cannabinoids are the primary compound in marijuana that deliver the medicinal and relaxing effects. There are approximately 80 different types of known cannabinoids; the most notable is THC (Tetrahydrocannabinol). Some other notable cannabinoids are CBD (Cannabidiol), CBC (Cannabichromene), and CBG (Cannabigerol).

Some clubs will test their products and will list the test results; this tells you the strength of a particular cannabinoid in that strain. Most frequently they test for THC and CBDs. This is one indicator of the quality of the medication and it can be helpful when you're looking for a particular type of relief from your medicine. For instance, a high CBD strains are particularly good at helping with anxiety, stress and nausea.

As the federal government allows studies to finally be performed on marijuana that I'm sure they will discover what each cannabinoid provides patients. One may be great for anxiety; another may provide superior relief for those need an appetite stimulant. Only in depth studies will give us this information and the federal government has consistently stood in the way of these studies and further understanding of this wonderful, natural drug. Once the federal government is shamed into finally removing marijuana from the Schedule 1 drug list, pharmaceutical companies will likely utilize these studies to make medications from marijuana that they can sell to consumers.

Q: What is THC?

A: THC stands for Tetrahydrocannabinol is the crystaline, and the primary active compound in marijuana. THC has many positive effects medicinally. First and foremost, it provides mild to moderate pain management. Other side effects are appetite stimulation, relaxation, reduced aggression and anger as well as providing some mild antioxidant effects.

Q: What is CBD?

A: CBD is another cannabinoid in cannabis called Cannabidiol. CBDs have been found to be particularly good at treating those with pain, nausea, inflammation, anxiety, depression, and stress as well as inhibiting cancer growth. An Oct, 2013 study by the University of California showed that high CBD marijuana not only helps to control flare ups of Crohn's and Ulcerative Colitis but that it actually can cure some patients.

Studies have shown that cannabis high in CBD attacks cancer cells in breast, skin, brain, leukemia and thyroid cancers and even inhibits growth of tumors.

CBDs will lessen the psychoactive effects of THC, making it an excellent medication for daytime use. High CBD strains will still have some psychoactive effects but they will generally leave you feeling more uplifted and clear headed than a low CBD strain.

Q: What is CBC?

A: Also called Cannabichromene. CBC's have been shown to play a roll in anti-inflammatory, anti-viral and pain management effects.

Q: What is CBG?

A: CBG, also called Cannabigerol, is known to help relieve intra-ocular pressure. This special cannabinoid is also thought to possess anti-microbial properties as well as being a good sedative. Anti-microbial is defined as killing or inhibiting the growth of microorganisms such as mold, fungus and bacterial infections.

Q: Is medical cannabis organic?

A: Because the U.S. Department of Agriculture is the only entity allowed to label a product organic, and because marijuana is illegal federally, there is no marijuana that can officially be called or labeled organic. Most medical cannabis is grown with organic standards and organic materials. Unless your grower is Clean Green Certified (http://bit.ly/1fLYCuh) you will have to rely on growers and clubs to tell you whether or not a strain was grown with organic standards. Clean Green is a private business that is not backed by the U.S. Department of Agriculture, as is common with organic food certifications. This means that Clean Green cannot label marijuana 'organic'. Clean Green has a set of rules and regulations that growers must follow that are similar to those that the federal government would label organic.

"Organic crops and products are certified by private agencies through the U.S. Department of Agriculture — a program developed after decades of advocacy by organic farmers and their allies. Pot — medicinal or otherwise — need not apply."[19]

Since many clubs do not grow or produce their own

---

[19] "Medical Marijuana Can't Be Organic, Which Troubles Growers - Los Angeles Times." Accessed September 14, 2013. http://articles.latimes.com/2011/aug/20/business/la-fi-organic-pot-

products, verifying for sure whether or not they are organic is slightly more difficult. Even if a club grows everything organically and sustainably they cannot call themselves organic.

According to Matthew Cohen, executive director of Northstone, a Ukiah-based delivery service; they may label their pot as "grown with organic nutrients sustainably"; but they cannot list it as organic. [20]

If you're concerned about it, ask your club if they ask growers to explain their grow methods and if they grow with organic nutrients. If they can't tell you then you should find another club.

Q: What kind of marijuana works best for my condition?

A: Everyone is different and therefore how you are affected by a particular strain is also slightly different. Just as we all prefer different foods or react to medications differently, we all will prefer different strains for the effects, how they taste and even how they smell is personal preference. I like the smell of fruity strains while others may prefer more skunky smelling marijuana. I prefer *indica*-leaning strains while a close friend of mine prefers *sativas,* though we both utilize all types of strains.

It's good to read about the differences between *indica, sativa*

---

[20] "Is Your Medical Marijuana Organic?" Accessed September 14, 2013.
http://blogs.sfweekly.com/thesnitch/2011/08/is_your_medical_marijuana_orga.php.

and hybrids but ultimately the best way to find out what effects you like is to try out different strains. I have several strains that I like to keep on hand. *Indicas* work better for sleeping. *Sativas* seem to help with headaches. I have *sativas, indicas* and hybrids that are all great for pain but some are better for daytime use while others are extremely sedative, and therefore are better for use before bedtime. Read ahead for more information on the different types of strains to get a good idea of where to start. If you're able to, buy a small amount of several different strains to start.

Q: What's the difference between indoor and outdoor marijuana?

A: This is a source of heated debate amongst growers, clubs and patients. Some claim indoor is better because of stable conditions; others claim outdoor is better due to the larger spectrum of light given off by the sun. Personally, I've had great outdoor and indoor medications. The price of outdoor medications has crashed in the last few years in California, making quality medication more affordable.

Some strains grow better outdoor than indoor and vice versa so you may find some strains are primarily available during outdoor growing months.

Outdoor strains are more susceptible to pests, bug larva, mold, mildew and even bird poop. It's exposed to the outdoors and therefore anything in the environment, the soil, etc., is possibly in the plant. Some people will only use indoor medication because they feel it's healthier and less likely to cause issues with allergies.

If you don't live in a warm area, you may have only one growing season. This means that if you are using only outdoor marijuana you will need to either buy or grow a large amount and try to store it and smoke aging bud while waiting for the next years crop or you will need to supplement this with indoor. If you're lucky enough to live where you can grow outdoor year-round, or even several months of the year, then you can likely get good outdoor marijuana for great prices all year.

Indoor marijuana is grown in stable, controlled temperatures and conditions. It can be grown year round and so you can get the same strain, from the same club, from the same grower, all year. Because the conditions are controlled, the quality is generally similar in each batch.

Bottom line is that you will find excellent outdoor and great indoor marijuana here in California.

Q: How can I find reasonably priced marijuana?

A: Over the years I have learned some of the best ways to get the best deals and to stretch my dollar. Hopefully these tips will help you save a bit along the way.

- Vaporize your plant and concentrated cannabis. Vaporizing is a much more efficient use of marijuana and will make it last much longer than if you smoke it. A good vaporizer will pay for itself in a very short time.

  - Use and make edibles. A $10 Cheeba Chew (http://bit.ly/GCVIce) has four strong doses in it that will last all day. $2.50 for a day of medication is a great price. If you make your own edibles, you can stretch your dollar even further. I used a quarter ounce of high quality outdoor marijuana to make enough marijuana butter (canna-butter) to make a full batch of brownies (I used a box of brand name brownies that need butter or oil to make them) and I ended up with nearly 30 very strong doses of small brownies. This cost $25 for the marijuana and about $5 for the stick of butter and the box of brownies, taking my cost of this down to $1 per dose/per day. Not bad!

- Buy low cost, great quality outdoor strains for a fraction of what you pay for indoor of a similar quality. I've found several places that have amazing outdoor for $100 per ounce. Compare this to the $300 per ounce for indoor pot and you're getting a great deal.

- Don't just settle on one club, try out many of them and find the best medicine at the best price by shopping around. Every time you visit a new club you will typically get a free gift; this can range from a small thing of kief, $10 in credit in the club, and even as much as a free 1/8 oz.

- Many clubs offer specials, coupons, and other types of deals. Check leafly.com or weedmaps.com and the club's website for deals, updates, menus, potency testing and pricing.

- Join the email list of your club so that when they do offer a deal you know about it.

- Buy in bulk. Typically, the more you buy, the less it costs by weight. If you can afford to buy more at a time this will save you some money.

- Pay someone else to grow your crop. Some growers will grow a crop for a specific patient. This will cost you less than purchasing marijuana from clubs but more than growing the medicine yourself.

- Consider growing your own marijuana, whether it's outdoor or indoor; a small investment up front will save you a ton of money. Cannabis is not particularly difficult to grow and there are countless videos on youtube.com, books on amazon.com and free guides online regarding growing marijuana that anyone can do it. A small investment up front can produce a lot of marijuana in the future.

Q: How do I prepare marijuana buds for smoking or vaporizing?

A: When you buy from a club you should receive buds that have already been processed, meaning someone has removed the larger stems and unusable material. Quality marijuana will not have seeds in it but if you happen to get some with seeds, remove those as well.

Remove any remaining stems as these are not something you want to smoke or vaporizer. You can pull apart the buds/flowers with your hands but this is not the recommended way to break up marijuana today because the trichomes that contain a lot of the medicinal value will stick to your fingers and even get knocked off while you are separating it with your hands.

The better way to do this is to purchase a grinder. Grinders make it fast and easy to grind up plant material and they grind it up in small pieces so that when you burn or vaporize the material you will get the most THC out of it. Grinders are a small, handheld device; they are much like a spice grinder and they usually twist back and forth or have a crank on the top to turn the device. It usually will have many metal sharp teeth inside to cut up the marijuana.

Q: What types of grinders are available and what works best?

A: You will find a huge variety of grinders available at your local pipe shop (also referred to as a head shop) and online. They range from $10 for a cheaper plastic model to over a $100 for a hand machined aluminum brand name model. I have owned both brand name and more generic models. I don't recommend the plastic models as they don't clean up as nicely, nor do they do as good of a job grinding up the plant material.

Some grinders are two parts and they grind the material and you shake or brush the material out afterwards. These work well but I find the trichomes build up quite badly in these types of grinders as they have no place to go; this causes the grinder to get gunked up quickly.

I prefer a grinder with a few sections, one that has kief screen and collection area on the bottom. It seems to collect a lot of kief as well as providing a place for the kief to go so the grinder just does not get as sticky and messy as fast. As a bonus, you get to use the kief in the bottom to give whatever bud you have a boost. You can sprinkle the kief on top of other plant material or press it into discs with a kief press and then vaporize or smoke it.

I have found a particularly good grinder that is inexpensive and of a good quality. I've had mine for several months and it's still working great. The grinders available at the pipe shops have a much higher markup on them.

If you want to search for a grinder online I highly recommend you buy one from a site that has reviews. There are plenty of them on eBay, but most of them are junk and it's hard to tell the good from the bad with the lack of reviews.

My favorite low cost, crank handle type grinder is one I bought on Amazon.com. It's of pretty good construction. You can buy it here:

http://amzn.to/19r6ajG

Q: How do I clean a grinder without losing the trichomes?

A: If you bought an aluminum grinder (most of them are aluminum) I recommend first putting it in the freezer for about 30-60 minutes. You will want to scrape the trichomes onto a plate, bowl or other dish. It is best to use a glass dish or plate so the stuff doesn't stick to it easily.

Holding the grinder over the plate/bowl then take a small tool or a small hard bristled brush, toothpicks or even a small flathead screwdriver and scrape the stuff off of the grinder. Because it's cold it will come of more easily. You can collect all the material off of the plate and use it boost your bud by sprinkling on it.

To further clean your grinder, see my question below about great ways to clean your pipes. This will work on your grinder.

Q: What is the process for smoking marijuana?

A: If you're a beginner to marijuana and you don't already smoke cigarettes, then you may want to try vaporizing because smoke can be irritating to the lungs. It's just healthier to vaporize rather than smoke marijuana and it's less expensive.

Having that over with, some people may want to smoke it. It has a slightly different effect than vaporizing so some people will switch between vaporizing and smoking.

Once the material is broken up, it can be smoked by rolling it in a joint, smoking it in a pipe or a water pipe (also called a bong).

I would avoid the use of 'blunts'. Hip-hop culture has made blunts extremely popular amongst younger smokers. They use tobacco leaf rolling paper products to roll large joints. They come in different flavors and are even sweet at times. Not only is this wasteful of your product, with the majority of your THC just going into the air, but you can also get addicted to nicotine if you use these papers regularly. The papers will mask any flavors of the strains you may enjoy, and nicotine is an addiction that's difficult to kick.

If you want to smoke marijuana in a joint just get regular

rolling papers. If you don't know how to roll you can purchase a roller for around $5-$10 that makes rolling cigarette looking joints quick and easy. Rollers and papers come in different sizes so make sure you buy the right size papers for your roller.

You can also smoke marijuana in a pipe. Smoking marijuana in a pipe is best done by using the cornering method of smoking. The idea is to only burn a small portion of the bowl of green pot rather than placing the flame in the center of the bowl. Once the flame hits a small section of the green marijuana, it will burn up nearly all the available cannabinoids in that area. Smoking marijuana is the least efficient way to extract and use all the THC in that much of it is just burned up and released in to the air. 'Cornering' is considered good pot etiquette when sharing with other people.

Q: What kinds of pipes are used to smoke marijuana?

A: Marijuana pipes come in all shapes, sizes and materials. The most popular type of pipe is the hand blown glass pipes you will find at pipe shops and online. These are popular because they don't get hot, they clean up easily, you can see the smoke as it enters the pipe and they can be beautiful pieces of art. I prefer buying these at the pipe shops because you can feel the weight and quality of the pipe at the shop. A nice pipe will not break as easily as a cheap, thin pipe. If they aren't blown at a consistent thickness, they will have weaknesses in them and they will break or chip easily. Most of these pipes have a choke hole in them that you place your thumb over and then release once the pipe is full of smoke.

THE CALIFORNIA MEDICAL MARIJUANA PATIENTS BOOK

You can also get water pipes to smoke through. These help cool the smoke as well as filter it through water. This has been shown to remove a small amount of toxins from the smoke; it also removes a small amount of THC as well. If you smoke, it's better to smoke it through a water pipe.

You will also find wood, metal and even mediums such as clay pipes. I have always preferred glass over the other mediums for pipes. You will find people who love each type of pipe. There are some things you just cannot make with glass that you can make with wood so you will find very different styles depending on the medium of the piece.

If you don't have a pipe and you don't want to smoke it in joint form you can easily make a pipe out everything from an apple to a tool.

There are many videos on how to make pipes, check them out here:

http://bit.ly/15PhULZ

Q: How do I clean pipes and other marijuana accessories?

A: The pipe shops love to sell this stuff that claims to clean your pipes easily. It's expensive and it's not that great. Many times this stuff is just rubbing alcohol with large salt chunks in it; you put in the pipe and shake up. I don't like it and have found a method that works really great.

I have a few ways that I think work well. I use these methods to clean glass, metal and even silicone parts.

My favorite cleaner is Stain Solvent. This stuff cleans

anything! It will clean everything from your grout, to an old hat to your pipe and it's non-toxic and safe. Just soak for a few hours and then rinse, if it's really dirty then you may have to soak it twice.

Stain Solvent on Amazon

http://amzn.to/1f9FJRB

You can likely get these cleaners at your local home store as well.

Another method is using a high concentrate (90%) rubbing alcohol. You can also just let this soak and it will likely clean most of the material out of your pipe or grinder. I use rubbing alcohol on grinders, as it seems to work very well. Just let it soak and then scrub them with a toothbrush.

It's always good to have pipe cleaners and small bottle brushes on hand to clean hard to reach areas in your pipes and equipment.

The key to painless cleaning is soaking your accessories overnight. I have a small bucket and will fill up the glass piece with either alcohol or the Stain Solvent mixture and let it sit under the sink overnight.

Q: Smoking marijuana is smelly, how can I hide the smell of it indoors?

A: The easiest way is to vaporize your marijuana, as it has very little smell in comparison to smoked pot. If you're a smoker and that's not going to change, then you can try some of these tips.

THE CALIFORNIA MEDICAL MARIJUANA PATIENTS BOOK

It is much easier to cover up the smell of marijuana if you choose a smaller space to smoke it in such as a bedroom, bathroom or any enclosed area. Larger areas such as open basements or large rooms with big vaulted ceilings will be more difficult to quickly cover up smells.

Another trick that works is to smoke in a bathroom. Turn on the shower or water on hot and let it run to steam up the room a bit, blow the smoke into the steam.

You can use incense and candles, they do an okay job of covering it up but if you ask me, it's a dead giveaway. Pot smokers love incense.

One thing people have used is a tube (also called a sploof) that you can exhale the smoke through like a filter. You can create one by using the center of a toilet paper roll and taking several dryer sheets and stuffing them into one end. Take tape and put a little over the one end so they don't fall out. Exhale your smoke through the tube and it will filter out nearly all the smell. You still have to deal with the smoke coming out of your bowl or off of your joint and this can still create an incredible amount of smell and smoke.

Here is a good tutorial on how to make a sploof.
http://bit.ly/16nP0NP

Purchase some Ozium air neutralizer. This is by far the best air neutralizer/freshener that you will find, and it does a better than average job of covering up and removing the smell from the air. It's really strong so don't use it like other air fresheners. Spray one short spray in to the middle of your room after smoking. Make sure to put away any marijuana or food before spraying Ozium, it probably would not taste good on your marijuana nor is it safe for consumption.

You can also use a power hitter or smokeless bottle. When I was in college you could buy these at the pipe shops and you may still be able to but you can easily and cheaply make your own at home with any squeeze type bottle with the right top. The idea is to use a squeeze type bottle (mustard bottles work well) and to fit a joint to the inside of the bottle. Then cut a small hole in the bottle to use as a choke. If possible, it is good to attach a silicone tube (food grade) inside to put the end of the joint in it. Light the joint, put it in the underside of the lid, screw the lid on and squeeze.

Since this description is not sufficient to make your own, here is a great thread on creating a bottle for yourself.

http://bit.ly/1e576cG

This person has made one out of a water bottle.

http://bit.ly/15iRjVd

Here is a video of a guy using another homemade power hitter.

http://bit.ly/1fVXJAn

Q: How can I make sure I don't smell like marijuana after smoking it?

A: Vaporizing marijuana is the best way to not smell like pot. While it still has some smell, it just will not stick to your body and clothing in the way that smoking marijuana sticks to you.

The first thing you can do is do not smoke marijuana in small enclosed areas such as cars. If you have a safe and discrete place, it is best to smoke outdoors so the smoke doesn't stay around you.

If you smoke indoors, try to use an exhaust fan or a fan in the window. You can use dryer sheets on a fan or over a vent that exhausts outside to cover up the smell. Blow the smoke away from you. Do not carry roaches or burnt marijuana on your person.

When you're finished smoking you should wash your hands. If you smoked in an enclosed area you likely have the smell all over you. Use a nice smelling lotion and put lotion on your arms, hands, face, etc. Brush your teeth or chew some gum. Top all of this off with a spritz or splash of your favorite cologne or perfume.

If you were in a really small area, if there was a lot of smoke or the exposure was long, you may want to change your clothing.

Q: What is vaporizing or vaping?

A: Vaporizing works by gradually heating the plant material or concentrate to a temperature of 356° F - 400° F; this process extracts the active cannabinoids for inhalation while avoiding the toxic and carcinogenic by-products. Combusting (burning) material begins around 450° and the carcinogenic elements are created during the combustion process. The THC and other cannabinoids begin to vaporize at about 350°. This essentially separates the cannabinoids from the plant material while avoiding combusting and the creation of the junk you don't want in your lungs.

Vaporizing is much less irritating to the throat and lungs and since combusting (burning) the plant matter is largely what creates the carcinogens, you avoid delivering tar and bad things to your respiratory system while still getting the THC.

When you smoke marijuana you are inhaling approximately 15% THC and 85% other non-cannabinoid gases. Vaporizing strips nearly all of that junk you don't want out; depending on the efficiency of the vaporizer vapor has been tested to contain between 35% - 96% cannabinoids; that's all medicine.

Smoking marijuana tends to combust it at much higher temperatures than necessary, thus destroying much of the cannabinoids in the process. This means that you will extract and use more of the cannabinoids when vaporizing than smoking; this makes vaporizing more affordable.

Q: What's the process for vaporizing marijuana?

A: How you prepare the plant material is similar to how you prepare it for smoking. Each vaporizer will have different instructions and different amounts you must use in it for it to function at its peak. One vaporizer may require you to completely top off the chamber that holds the material while others will allow you to put in what you want. For the process please check the individual instructions of each vaporizer.

The key is to grind up your plant material in a small grind, the smaller the grind the better when vaporizing. Each vaporizer will have a compartment to put your material. It's very important not to over pack your material. It should be packed but not too tight. You want air to be able to pass through the material for plant material vaporizers.

Q: What does vaporized marijuana smell like?

A: Vaporized marijuana may still put off a marijuana smell but it's likely to be much more subtle than when you smoke it. The smell it puts off great depends on the vaporizer and whether you are vaporizing plant material or a form of concentrate. Plant material will put off more of a smell but it's still quite mild. It still smells like marijuana but instead of the typical burned smell it's more of a natural, fresh marijuana smell; it's not nearly as recognizable to non-marijuana consumers. It's so mild that it's easily covered up.

The smell of vaporized marijuana will disappear much more quickly than that of smoked pot. A candle or a spray of any air freshener will likely be a good cover. The O-Phos and most other pen vaporizers create a pretty subtle smell when I vaporize full-melt wax.

Q: What kinds of vaporizers are available?

A: There are literally hundreds, probably even thousands of different vaporizers in the world. People build them at home while others buy them.

There are two main types of vaporizers on the market, conduction and convection. Most vaporizers have some elements of both conduction and convection but they will usually be more one type than the other.

Conduction vaporizers heat the material directly by the material sitting directly on the heated surface (much like a bread machine heats from all sides). Conduction vaporizers generally work better with a smaller grind of the plant material and they can at times slightly combust the material. They may also have a tendency to cook the material unevenly and continuously, thus using up the THC content even when you're not inhaling through it. Often times you will need to shake the vaporizer or open the chamber and stir up the material in order to extract the maximum medicinal value.

I'm not a huge fan of some conduction vaporizers as I don't think the material tastes as good as long. I owned the Iolite for a while and I really only liked the taste of the first two hits, after that the taste leaned towards a very baked, used flavor that is not nearly as pleasant.

You shouldn't rule out all conduction vaporizers, more modern and recent designs have been engineered to eliminate or at least minimize these negatives and so you will find both types of vaporizers can be excellent.

Convection vaporizers heat the material by having a heating chamber separate from the chamber where the plant material is stored; hot air is then passed over and through the plant material evenly. Convection vapes are generally much more efficient designs, have better temperature controls, and they avoid combustion by having no or little direct contact with the heated surface.

THE CALIFORNIA MEDICAL MARIJUANA PATIENTS BOOK

Some vaporizers use cartridges, some use bags, while others have one chamber that must be filled, emptied and cleaned. Others use atomizers or cartridges that allow you to load a certain amount of concentrated cannabis and take a couple of hits all the way to hundreds of hits. Some have reusable cartridges while others are disposable and must be thrown out and replaced once spent.

There are vaporizers that must be plugged in for power, some that use batteries that you must recharge and others that run on butane. Some vaporizers require the use of a torch lighter. There are portable vaporizers and home vaporizers. Some are pretty large; such as the Volcano vaporizer while others are pocket or pen sized and will easily fit in your pocket.

Some vaporizers have a longer heat up time (Underdog) and are meant to stay on all day and therefore are available all the time and then others are ready in seconds (O-Phos or BHOLT).

You may be able to control the temperature down to the degree on one model (Volcano digital), others just have a dial (Volcano classic), some may have several heat settings that are just ordered 1, 2, 3, or Low, Medium, High (Solo or Pax) that are pre-set and another may have a single temperature without any adjustment (O-Phos or BHOLT).

I lean towards convenient, easy to clean, portable vaporizers but I have some that need to be plugged in and others that are more difficult to clean. Choosing vaporizers is just as personal as choosing a strain. My best friend has vaporizers that she would call her favorites that I'm not interested in because they take more work than I want to put in when vaporizing. There are some of vaporizers that require the use of torch lighters and I'm a klutz on a good day, while completely clear headed. Give me a torch lighter while ill and feeling fuzzy headed, and I'm guaranteed to burn myself (best case), or catch something on fire (worst case). :) I've used these types of vapes and these can offer some of the most incredible hits of vapor (truly a one hit experience) that are extremely potent. You can see how this type of vaporizer may not work for some people but it may be the next person's favorite.

Q: What is the effect of vaporizing at different temperatures?

A: Vaporizing at lower temperatures will typically produce a thinner vapor; this thinner vapor contains less cannabinoids than vapor created at higher temperatures. The thicker vapor contains more cannabinoids. Some people will vaporize at a temperature as high as 420°; this will create a very thick, cannabinoid-rich vapor but it will not taste as good as if you vaporize your material at a lower temperature.

With one of my log vaporizers I usually vaporize somewhere around 375° as this gives me a nice thick vapor while still letting me enjoy the delicate flavors of the strain. Vaporizing at this level doesn't mean I lose out on the extra cannabinoids that I could get at a higher temperature; it just means that I will vaporize that material for a longer session in order to extract all of it's cannabinoids. In the end; you get the same amount of medication from that same plant material.

THE CALIFORNIA MEDICAL MARIJUANA PATIENTS BOOK

Every vaporizer is different and not all of them list temperatures. One vaporizer may produce a good vapor at 375° for you and your other vaporizer may have to be set to 385° to get the same effect. Many vaporizers that list temperature are showing the heater temperature, not the temperature of the air as it passes over the plant.

Play with the temperatures; it is a personal preference. Beginners may like lower temperatures until they are used to vaporizing and inhaling something.

Q: Where can I buy vaporizers?

A: You can buy vaporizers at your local pipe shop (also called a head shop), some clubs sell them, and you can buy them online. I haven't bought vaporizers from clubs because the ones I've seen in clubs are usually generic vaporizers made in China. These typically have a huge price markup; they usually have no brand, little or no warranty, and it will likely be difficult to find parts.

I prefer to buy most of my vaporizers online and I prefer vapes that I can research via reviews. Some vaporizers will only be at a set price; whether you get them online or in a shop. If the price at the local shop is the same or even close to the price online then I opt to support the local shop. If I can't get it locally or it's significantly cheaper then I buy it online. There are so many vaporizers on the market right now that you will find that many are only available online.

That doesn't mean you should write off buying from head shops offer one thing that online purchasing cannot, instant gratification. Also, I've always bought pipes in head shops because I could hold the piece and get an idea of the quality. I don't feel I need to do this with vaporizers as I usually buy a brand that I can research and so I already know what to expect from the product.

Do a Google search for the vaporizer when you want to compare pricing. This will give you an idea of who is offering that vaporizer and at what prices. Once you find a place you want to purchase a vaporizer from then Google for coupons for that site by Googling the website name and the word coupon or code. Example: 'delta9vapes.com coupon' or 'delta9vapes.com code'

Q: What vaporizers would I recommend?

A: I can recommend some vaporizers that I have experience with already but understand that there are hundreds of vaporizers available for sale today and I'm only going to cover a few here. You should check out www.fuckcombustion.com for a more complete view of vaporizers and their reviews.

Solo

www.arizer.com - bit.ly/15UYDGJ

The Solo is my favorite at-home, battery-powered vaporizer for buds/flowers. It uses a beveled glass stem with a screen about 1/2" from one end, leaving a small compartment to pack with ground up flower material. It heats up in a couple of minutes and has heat settings of 1-7. It runs on a rechargeable internal battery that lasts for about a dozen 15-minute sessions. I love this vaporizer because it's uses a small amount of ground up buds and it goes a long way.

THE CALIFORNIA MEDICAL MARIJUANA PATIENTS BOOK

This vaporizer makes my buds go so much further than when I used to combust them. I love the convenience of moving around the house. It doesn't cook the marijuana and give it that baked taste that I don't really like. Cleaning and maintenance is minimal; just clean the stem by soaking it in rubbing alcohol.

O-Phos

www.w9tech.com - bit.ly/19WxRxh

The O-Phos is a cartridge-based full-melt concentrate vaporizer and it's amazing. It's a little larger than a pen and easily fits in my pocket or bag. The O-Phos charges via a standard USB charger and holds a charge for a long time. I charge mine about every three to four days and I'm very happy with the battery life. The O-Phos is based on cartridges which means that it requires nearly no cleaning. This is also one of it's drawbacks because you must replace the cartridges after use. The good news is that a cartridge lasts a long time. One cartridge will technically hold 1 gram of full-melt concentrate, though I have loaded up to 1.5 grams on a couple of them. You load it with approximately 60% of a gram of wax. Once that is used up (you will get a metallic taste and no vapor) then you add the rest of your gram. I've used an old cart to just toss in a bunch of leftover waxes and it took another half (1/2) gram. This pen vape makes my concentrates last uber long. I can use one cartridge and a gram for a full month and I use my O-Phos everyday. The cartridges cost $10 each but for the convenience of no cleaning mixed with how far this stretches your concentrate dollars, I love it.

T. OLIVER

BHOLT (Pronounced 'bolt')

www.bholtvape.com - bit.ly/1d8pq78

The BHOLT is a beast of a wax vaporizer as it will deliver monster hits of thick vapor from the moment you load it. It's a pen style but it's more bulky than the O-Phos. The BHOLT charges via USB and holds a charge for a full day, though since I do not use this all day long mine seems to need a charge every few days. It is the ultimate quick relief, fast-track to feeling the effects of marijuana. It uses a consumable atomizer with a small ceramic bowl inside. This vaporizer is perfect for loading your favorite strain and taking several hits and then loading another strain. It's easy to load and requires almost no cleaning. It delivers such large hits that it's an entirely different vape from that of the other pen style vapes. I use this when I am exceptionally ill or when I have friends over who want to get really, really stoned. It's inexpensive and it's made entirely in US, each atomizer is handmade by the owner and his helpers. The atomizers are $20 each but they last for a really long time. While no-where near as smelly as smoking marijuana, the vapor is so thick that it puts off a decent amount of fresh marijuana smell. I don't recommend this one as a discrete way of medicating in public though it would work great for travel when you've got a place to medicate in private, such as a hotel room. Get one, they are awesome.

Illadelph Hot Hit Slide w/ Flex Glass Mini Rig

www.aqualabtechnologies.com - http://bit.ly/1gisxdZ
www.errld.com - http://bit.ly/1f9Dmfl

Generally I avoid flame-powered vapes because I am accident prone but I could not resist this one. The Hot Hit Slide from Illadelph is a beautiful piece of glass. I use this with the Flex Glass Mini Rig. To use this as a wax vaporizer you will need to buy a glow rod and torch lighter. The glow rod is essentially a stick of glass with a slightly bubbled end. You put the wax in the bowl and then torch the glow rod until it's a hot orange and then place it in the bowl and take a hit. This gives the best tasting wax hits that I have ever tried and it's all glass. It's more work and involves using a flame but the hits from this are incredibly strong. If you want a really fast way to medicate, this is truly a one-hit system. The first time I tried it I honestly felt like I had consumed a strong edible.

I use the 14mm female Flex Mini Rig with my BHOLT as well. These pieces use a standard of 14mm or 18mm connections so be sure to buy the correct size. There are even adapter pieces available so you can use the Solo with the Flex Mini Rig. If you like glass, you should consider investing in the Flex or something like it.

Q: How much do vaporizers cost?

A: Quality does somewhat correlate with price but it really depends on what you buy, and where you buy it. If you buy cheap vapes sold by most clubs for around $90-$100, you're probably getting a $20-$35 product.

If you really want to buy something like this then you should look on eBay; you will find an abundance of low-cost vaporizers that are likely similar to what they sell in many clubs, and at a fraction of the cost.

T. OLIVER

Here is a search on eBay for pen vapes.

http://bit.ly/1i6Gb02

You can also try out this link for a general eBay search on vaporizers:

http://bit.ly/1cKE9lK

You can buy 510 threaded pen vapes and different atomizers online. This is a great way to try out all types of atomizers with one battery base. I recommend getting a high quality vaporizer base like the BHOLT and then buying atomizers, as the batteries on eBay are no where near the quality of the BHOLT. They don't hold a charge as long and they probably won't last as long overall.

Spend wisely and do your homework and you can get really great vaporizer for very little money.

My favorite concentrate pen vaporizer is the O-Phos (it's big sister is the Omnicrom) and I paid about $70 for when it while it was on sale. Vaporizers will range from $20 for a smaller, cheaper vape up to $700 for the BMW of vaporizers; the Digital Volcano. I've owned a Digital Volcano and I've owned lower end vaporizers and the price was not what determined me favoring that device. You can find great vaporizers at nearly every price point.

Q: Will one vaporizer work for all of my needs?

A: I'm sure there are people who are able to get by on a single vaporizer, but that's not me. Someone who only needs to consumer marijuana in the evening, doesn't travel

THE CALIFORNIA MEDICAL MARIJUANA PATIENTS BOOK

and doesn't want to use it unless they are at home may be ok with a single vaporizer. I currently have several vaporizers, three of those that I use regularly. My friends who prefer vaporizing to smoking also tend to have more than one vaporizer. One of my friends has a collection of vaporizers because she likes having them for different materials and different situations.

I lean towards convenient and simple vaporizers that don't require a lot of cleaning or work. I also don't really care for those vaporizers that require me to use torch lighters or to work with really hot things like hot nails. This is mainly because I like convenience and I'm a little accident-prone. I don't want to be medicating and having to think about not burning the crap out of myself with a red-hot nail. Many of those types of vaporizers have given me some of the best hits of vapor I've ever received (thanks to my friends who buy them) but for my daily use they just don't work for me.

If your aim is to vaporize most of the time rather than smoke, then I recommend you buy more than one vaporizer. Even if you own the Digital Volcano, it doesn't help you when you need to vaporizer away from home and I wouldn't use it for concentrates. I didn't fully embrace vaporizing until I had at least two vaporizers that I really liked.

I have a pen vaporizer that I love and use regularly; it heats instantly and only requires loading concentrates every so often. It's very portable and discrete and runs off of a rechargeable battery.

I have a log vaporizer that I leave in my garage for use on

weekends. It has to be plugged into an outlet and takes about 25 minutes to reach vaporizing temperatures. It's extremely efficient and makes my plant material last for a really long time. I use a small amount of marijuana and can get many hits of vapor off of it. You can leave it plugged in 24 hours a day and just turn down the temperature and use it as an aromatherapy unit when not vaporizing with it.

I have a battery powered, portable plant material vaporizer that is very similar to my log vaporizer except that it's portable. I would say this is my second favorite vaporizer because of its convenience and ease of hiding it.

You can see how someone might own several vaporizers in order to meet all of their needs.

Q: Does smoking and vaporizing marijuana have the same biological effects?

A: Vaporizing and smoking are similar in that both methods provide rapid onset delivery, meaning you will feel the effects and get relief nearly instantly. Both methods allow for easy proper dosing.

Todays vaporizers are very efficient and are likely to extract the most cannabinoids from your marijuana in compared to smoking. Marijuana smoke contains up to 85-90% of toxins and chemicals and only 10-15% of THC and cannabinoids. Vapor can contain up to 96% cannabinoids, making it much purer medication.

A 2007, University of California San Francisco study found that vaporized cannabis contains the biological effects as smoking cannabis but without the toxins and carcinogens of burning marijuana.

I find the effects of vaporizing to be very similar to smoking, except I don't cough as much and I don't feel the negative effects on my lungs or throat the next day.

There are mild differences in the effects. Some users report vaporizing as being weaker or less intense than smoking, while others say it feels stronger when they vaporize. While it's true that vaporization extracts a much higher concentrate of THC and other cannabinoids than smoking it definitely feels different. Vaporizing seems to give a more heady, uplifting feeling than smoking. Smoking typically will deliver more of the body high effects, more couch-lock. This is why I will still occasionally smoke marijuana.

Q: Are there other benefits to vaporizing pot?

A: Saving money is the other great benefit of vaporizing marijuana. If you don't have unlimited funds for your marijuana (if only!) then you should consider vaporizing because it will save you a lot of money, particularly if you have a few vaporizers available to you for different situations and forms of pot.

Vaporizing is a much more efficient use of marijuana and makes it go much further. When I used to smoke marijuana, I went through it very quickly (at least it felt like I did!) and it was super expensive. Since switching to vaporizing both plant material and concentrates it lasts me a really long time. I can vaporize half of an average size bowl of marijuana for nearly 15 minutes in my handheld *Arizer Solo* vaporizer. That same amount would be burned up in one or two hits if

I were smoking it in a pipe. I will get very nice effects off of this one tiny bowl in a vaporizer but not feel much if I smoked the same amount. Some people may balk at the prices of vaporizers, but I can tell you from experience that they will quickly pay for themselves by getting much more THC out of the material.

Q: What is AVB and what can I do with it?

A: AVB stands for Already Vaped Bud or Already Been Vaporized, depending on whom you ask. AVB will still contain many cannabinoids and can still be used. Don't try to smoke it, it will taste terrible but you can cook it into foods and use it that way. This is the most frequent use of AVB.

CAUTION: Because AVB still contains active cannabinoids you should store this as securely as you would store any of your marijuana. Keep it in a safe place where children and pets cannot get to it.

Q: Is consuming medical marijuana edibles the same as smoking or vaporizing it?

A: Typically edibles will last much longer and feel stronger than if you smoke or vaporize marijuana; the effects can last up to several hours. When you eat marijuana your liver metabolism will process and destroy some of the THC and then form a very potent THC metabolite.

In my experience, edibles can be particularly great in dealing with severe pain and nausea as the potency is higher than when marijuana is smoked or vaporized. They are also great when you need to medicate once or discretely and have relief all day.

If you're a beginner with edibles you should start small and try stronger doses. While pot can reduce anxiety and stress it can also increase anxiety when it's in edible form, especially for beginners. This anxiety should decrease significantly as you become used to the effects of edibles and marijuana in general.

You should be cautious as to how much of an edible you take because taking too much can be unpleasant and overwhelming. When smoking and vaporizing you will feel the effects nearly immediately so using too much is unlikely. Edibles can take 20-120 minutes to take effect and this can cause patients to over medicate. It can't kill you (not even close) but you won't enjoy waiting for it to wear off. It can cause acute anxiety and even panic as well as making the medication last as much as 8-16 hours.

When consuming pot you should always test out a small amount first. If it's not strong enough, wait a day and try again with a slightly larger dose.

Q: What kinds of edibles are available?

A: Edibles come in three categories, oral absorption (absorbed through saliva), gastrointestinal absorption (absorbed in the stomach), and hybrid absorption (absorbed through both).

The most common edibles are absorbed through the gastrointestinal system. They take longer to take effect but they will typically last for 6-8 hours. Some of the most common of these include brownies, cookies, peanut butter cups, pastries, chocolates, chocolate bars, cupcakes, breads, caramel popcorn, pies, crisp cereal rice treats, peanut butter bars, peanut brittle, truffles, savory *Chex*-like mix, ice cream, ice cream sandwiches, capsules; some places even serve medicated pizza!

Orally absorbed edible effects tend to take effect quickly, but they also wear off quicker. Orally absorbed edibles include tinctures and hard candies.

Hybrids are absorbed through our stomachs and orally. These include things like suckers, hard candy, cotton candy, rock candy, powdered drinks, caramels, sodas and more.

There are so many different edibles available today that it's not possible to name them all here. If you can cook it, bake it, or mix it up someone can likely figure out a way to infuse marijuana into it, and the edible makers never fail to keep innovating.

Special diet? Not to worry. You can find sugar free, vegan, nut allergies, all-natural and even gluten-free edibles.

Can't find what you want? You can easily make it at home. There are countless recipes online for all sorts of medicated foods.

Q: How can you tell the strength of an edible? How much should I eat?

A: Every product is different and every person is going to react slightly different. Potency is affected greatly by the quality of the marijuana used to make the edible. As with buds or concentrates, edibles can be *sativa*, *indica* or hybrid.

Some products list the potency and dosage; yet you still need to take your tolerance level in to consideration when using these products. These numbers mean almost nothing to me or any other consumers because they only test for one or two compounds. When you consider the different tolerances, metabolisms and biological makeup of each person you can understand how we may all have different experiences with the same medication. A particular edible may be strong for one person and just right for another, even if they eat the exact same dose.

My first recommendation is that you ask the club employees about the dose a product. Many products will list a dose. I have found some of those listed doses to be low and some seem to be too high. When I ask a club employee for a dose recommendation I let them know my tolerance is low.

The best advice I can give you is to start small. If it lists a whole peanut butter cup as a dose and you've never tried them before, take a half of a cup. Don't make the mistake of doubling down (taking more) because it wasn't strong enough. This is another way people over-medicate on edibles. You are much better off waiting for that edible to completely wear off and try a full peanut butter cup on another day as edibles can be quite strong.

Q: How long will it take for me to feel the effects of an edible?

A: The form of the edible, the strain, how it's absorbed into your system, the quality of the plant used, your metabolism;

all of these can skew the time it takes for you to feel the medication and its full potency. Edibles also seem to have a peak; a section of time when the medication is at it's strongest. It will start out mild and then get more intense until it hit's its peak. I find edibles absorbed in the stomach to have a peak of couple of hours on average, after this point it just gradually wears off.

A good dose for me will last me anywhere from 4-6 hours. I don't like really strong doses of edibles because they tend to make me less functional than smoking or vaporizing. I prefer that I barely feel it and therefore my doses don't last long. If I happen to be extremely ill, or if I know I don't have to be functional and productive, then I may take a larger dose; these deliver more pain management but also more of the psychoactive effects as well. A full dose will typically last 6-8 hours on average.

Just like marijuana plants, edibles can be *sativa*, *indica* or a hybrid. Some edibles will be high in CBDs while others are high in THC. While *indica* leaning strains are great at pain management they make me want to sleep so I only take them when I'm very ill and at home or if it's late at night. I usually prefer either hybrid or *sativa* edibles as they don't make me as sleepy.

Q: I took an edible, should I take more if I don't feel it?

A: I can't stress enough that if you don't feel your first dose is strong enough; you should try to avoid consuming more edibles that day to make it stronger. It is better to smoke or vaporize other forms of marijuana to add to the affect of the edible. This allows you to slowly increase your dose.

THE CALIFORNIA MEDICAL MARIJUANA PATIENTS BOOK

Q: Where can I find the best edibles?

A: Just as with other forms of the medication, you will find different edibles at each club. There are some brands that are now recognizable in the edible business and you will find them multiple clubs. Some clubs make their own edibles, while others only carry products made by others. Test them out. Ask the club employees what they prefer and why. Ask them for edibles suited to your specific condition or symptoms.

Once I find a good edible I will stick with that brand and type. I prefer caramels and chocolate because they are easy to conceal and transport, they don't have a really strong marijuana flavor in comparison to some other edibles and they don't typically require refrigeration. I like peanut butter cups for use at home (they usually have to be refrigerated). Medicated honey with an *indica* strain is great in tea in the evening before bed. You will find what you like and what works for you. Someone else may say they hate caramels and chocolate.

Q: Can I make my own edibles?

A: Yes, you can make your own edibles, it's inexpensive and it's not that difficult either! Most people start out by making cannabis butter (also called canna-butter) and then baking and cooking with the butter in any recipe that takes butter or oil. You can also purchase cannabis butter from many clubs. It's easy to make and it generally doesn't cost much to make a lot of cannabis butter. In my experience, cannabis butter goes a long way and will make many doses.

I'm not going to go through all the steps here but it essentially involves getting trimmings or even high quality buds (the better the material, the stronger your edibles), run it through a food processor so it's chopped up and cook it in butter (sometimes with water) until the oil from the marijuana combines with the oil from the butter. Strain through cheesecloth or a nut bag (yes they are actually called that, used for making almond or nut based milks) or a sieve and chill. Check my links below for more in depth instructions and recipes.

Once you have some cannabis butter you can use it wherever you would use butter or oil. You can buy a box of brownies that calls for oil or butter and substitute the same amount of the cannabis butter or you can make homemade muffins.

Here are some links to some butter recipes:

The Weed Blog - Easy Marijuana Butter Recipe - http://bit.ly/196SlEX

The Stoners Cookbook - http://bit.ly/1e2YjYB

MarijuanaRecipes.com - Best CannaButter Recipe Video - http://bit.ly/1ghWN77

Q: Is there a pill or capsule form of marijuana?

A: There is an FDA approved pill form of synthetic THC, called Marinol. Marinol is synthesized in a lab rather than being extracted from the actual plant. It's expensive to manufacture and has a long manufacturing process. It does not have the same effect as natural THC. It's primarily prescribed to help with nausea and appetite loss and is generally only prescribed to AIDS and cancer patients.

I have tried Marinol twice and I found it to have a small fraction of the therapeutic effects of natural marijuana. Leave it to the U.S. Government to approve a synthetic lab-version of a drug that you can already get in a safe, natural form.

There are capsules on the market now that are natural forms of marijuana. These are not FDA approved, though I don't take comfort in much the FDA does these days. These are usually push-together capsules that have concentrated cannabinoids inside. Some of the capsules look a lot like vitamin E capsules; I love these, as they are easy to travel with discretely. Capsules can be purchased at various clubs, call around or look on leafly.com, weedmaps.com or the club websites and I'm sure you will find some. Capsules offer a great way to get a consistent dose each time, though if you find a certain brand to be too strong, it's difficult to impossible to break these up in to smaller doses.

Q: What is an *indica*?

A: *Indicas* originate from Morocco, Tibet and Afghanistan. *Indica* plants are generally a short, broad and full variety of plant with deep green, wide leaves. *Indicas* are good indoor plants as they are shorter than *sativas*. The plants take six to eight weeks to mature after flowering; *indicas* are generally known to produce more than *sativas* and given the short vegetation period, you can get a couple of harvests in the time you would harvest once for *sativa* strains.

Indica flavors range from skunky to cheesy, and even sometimes fruity. They generally provide a very heavy, full-body high that people associate with "couch-lock"; meaning all you want to do is sit and do something like watch TV or relax. You may feel lazy or lethargic or just extremely relaxed. It can make you very sleepy, which makes it great for insomnia.

Indicas tend to be more of a full body high and are extremely relaxing so they good for stress. They are great medicines for nausea, pain, stress, muscle relaxation, expectorant, appetite stimulate, intra-ocular pressure relief, spasms, spasms, headaches, seizures, anxiety, and sleep issues. *Indicas* are typically favored by patients with cancer, AIDS, severe nausea and glaucoma.

Q: What is a *sativa*?

A: *Sativas* originate from Columbia, Mexico, and Southeast Asia and Thailand. *Sativa* plants are usually tall and thin with a lighter green color leaf. *Sativa* strains tend to grow better outdoors as some have been known to grow over 20 feet tall; though the average is just over 13 feet. The plants take ten to sixteen weeks to mature after flowering; because of this long vegetation period *sativa* strains can sometimes produce a few ounces per plant to a pound (1 lb.) of marijuana buds. Outdoor plants will typically produce more than indoor.

The flavors usually range from fruity to sweet, sometimes with hints of lemon or even pepper. They generally provide a more functional effect that will be more cerebral and uplifting, so they are an excellent daytime medication.

THE CALIFORNIA MEDICAL MARIJUANA PATIENTS BOOK

Sativas tend to contain more THC (tetrahydrocannabinol) than *indicas* and yet they are usually less potent. They can make you feel energetic and social. *Sativas* are more likely to cause long conversations about nothing, along with lots of laughter and fun. They can be the cause of some excellent introspection along with a feeling of elation. *Sativa* strains are great for daytime use and for times when you have to be social while medicated.

Some *sativas* will offer ok pain relief and they are anti-inflammatory, antispasmodic and sedative. For some conditions, *sativas* are not sufficient for pain management but you can easily look at a great hybrid to get the effects of both *indicas* and *sativas*. They are particularly great at providing relief for depression and stress because it's stimulating and uplifting. It also acts as an expectorant, relaxes muscles, relieves headaches and helps with nausea as well as being an appetite stimulant.

Q: What is ruderalis?

A: *Cannabis ruderalis* is a third and less known sub-species of *Cannabis*. It originates from Russia and therefore is a very hardy plant that is resistant to disease and can grow in more extreme climates. Unlike sativa and *indica* sub-species that flower based on hours of light the *ruderalis* strains flower based on age; referred to as auto-flowering. It's typically used more in hemp (non-medical) production than medical use. Because it is so hardy it's sometimes crossed with *sativa* or *indica* strains to produce disease resistant or auto-flowering hybrids.

T. OLIVER

Q: What is a hybrid?

A: A hybrid is any strain that contains both *indica* and *sativa* strains. Hybrids can have the best of both strains and allow growers to achieve a certain effect and even to produce better looking, tasting and smelling strains. Fruity *sativas* crossed with sweeter *indicas* make up some really great flavors that almost taste like berries at times.

Some hybrid crosses will be a 50/50 cross of *indica* and *sativa* while others are considered sativa-dominant or *indica* dominant; also referred to as *sativa-indica* or *indica-sativa*. Patients looking for really great pain management that won't lock you to a couch for half of a day may favor an *indica-sativa* hybrid strain. If you need an appetite stimulant but you don't want something too uplifting because it's later in the day you could opt for a *sativa-indica* strain. There are literally thousands of hybrid strains on the market and new ones are being developed everyday, every strain will affect you in a different way.

I love hybrid strains and recommend you try out some straight *sativas* and *indicas*. If you find two you like, you can probably find a hybrid of it. Sometimes I will find strains that contain three of my favorite strains and they rarely disappoint.

Q: What is kush?

A: Kush is a subset of strains of *Cannabis indica*. It originates from India, Pakistan and Afghanistan. Kush strains are usually short and wide with large, shiny trichomes covering the buds and usually have a citrus or even lemon flavor.

Kush strains were imported into the United States in the 1960s and 1970s. The strong *indica* strains drastically shortened the flowering and vegetative stage, allowing marijuana to be grown further north and in cooler climates than ever before. It literally changed the future of marijuana production in the U.S. Kush is particularly popular and prevalent in California. OG (Ocean Grown) originated from Northern California in the Lake Tahoe area.

I personally love kush strains and find them particularly great at fighting pain and nausea.

Q: What is sinsemilla?

A: Sinsemilla is seedless marijuana. Nearly all marijuana you will buy today will be sinsemilla. You may see some marijuana that has seeds in it from Mexico or from new growers. If your marijuana has seeds you will need to remove them all before grinding up the marijuana for use. In the last few years of buying from clubs I once received some marijuana that had two seeds in the entire bottle.

Q: What is a concentrate?

A: Concentrates are just that, concentrated THC and other cannabinoids that contain little to no plant matter. They come in the form of kief, hash, waxes, budder and oils. There are many variations on these but for the most part these are the main types of concentrates that you will find at nearly any club. Just like the marijuana buds, these concentrates are made from *indica*, sativa and hybrid strains.

T. OLIVER

Concentrates can be smoked, vaporized, smoked with the marijuana bud, and used in edibles.

Q: What is kief?

A: Kief is the resin glands or trichomes of the marijuana plant. These resin glands contain a higher concentrate of the cannabinoids than the rest of the bud. Some marijuana flower grinders will have a kief collector at the bottom. As the kief accumulates in the bottom of the grinder, you can collect it and sprinkle it on your bud, vaporize it, or press it into hash cakes and use them at a later time.

I have a kief grinder and press, though kief not my favorite form of medication. I have used it to give a boost to my buds when I'm feeling particularly ill or nauseous. I prefer grinders with kief collectors as the kief has a place to go; whereas my grinder without a kief collector gets really gummed up and sticky. It seems like a waste to lose that kief.

Q: What is hash?

A: One form of hash or hashish is pressed kief; resin glands (trichomes). Kief and hash can be consumed by smoking, vaporizing, making edibles and more. It's compressed so it can range from soft to hard and colors can range from a light beige to almost black. There is also bubble melt hash that is purified with water. Bubble melt hash is usually sticky and tar like and ranges in color from green to black. There is also hash made by rubbing the plants on your hands to collect trichomes and then scrape them off. I tried hash while in Jamaica that was made in this fashion and it was pretty harsh to smoke. It's typically dark and has lots of plant material in it.

There are many kinds of hash; most are named based on where it was made or the method or both.

I personally find hash to be quite harsh unless it's vaporized. Many pen style vaporizers that use wax, budder and oil concentrates won't use hash as it contains too much plant material.

Q: What is budder?

A: Budder is a concentrated THC (previously referred to as stable wax or earwax) that has a very high THC content and is whipped up and is in solid, yellow chunks. Some budder concentrates can have as much as 98% THC content; much higher than any bud or plant in it's natural form. Budder can only be made from high quality, fresh, source material. Wax and earwax will be sticky and more paste like, true budder will not be sticky at all.

Budder is the highest quality and highest concentrated marijuana medication. This was originally developed out of Canada by a man now referred to as "The Budder King". His budder was rumored to have tested to be as high as 98% Cannabinoids. This is a 100% stable, high quality and typically will be very strong with great flavors. Budder will be more solid and formed in chunks and is generally a yellow color. There are many dispensaries who advertise budder when in fact they are selling a lower quality version of this that is generally called wax. Budder is difficult to make and it must be made with only high quality buds and plant material. [21]

Budders are made by whipping the extracts while purging out the chemicals. Whipping the concentrate while heating it adds air to the product causing it to 'whip' up as it's cooling. "100% stable" generally refers to the product being solid and holding together well while not easily changing form and without tackiness to the product.

Budder contains little to no toxins like molds, diseases, heavy metals and other chemicals left behind by fertilizers and pesticides, making it particularly great for patients with immune issues.

While I utilize nearly all of the different forms of medical marijuana, budder and wax are my favorite. I find it easy to transport and when vaporized it puts off little to no smell; making it particularly great for medicating discretely. Because it's so concentrated and strong you don't need to carry as much with you.

Q: What is wax?

A: Wax is a great high quality concentrate; also referred to as full-melt wax, or earwax. These can range from soft earwax (Where did you think it got its name?), to silly putty, even really soft like a creamy peanut butter and will be

---

[21] "Differences Between Wax and Budder - Concentrated Cannabis - WeedTRACKER." Accessed September 14, 2013. http://dispensaryweed.com/cannabis/topic/193441-differences-between-wax-and-budder/.

semi-stable meaning they will be somewhat tacky to the touch while holding together well. Waxes are made from the marijuana plant via solvent extraction just as budder. Some people have said that wax is just a failed version of making budder but it's really more about timing and proper heat being applied during purging.

You can smoke or vaporize wax or you can put it on top of ground up marijuana.

These are some of the strongest forms of medical marijuana and they are excellent for medicating quickly as you will generally use less of it than you would the marijuana bud. Good wax will typically contain 70-98% THC. Most marijuana buds will average 5% THC for low quality outdoor buds to 27% THC for top shelf buds. (You're not likely to find buds that low in THC in most California clubs.)

"According to Animal New York's Matt Harve it's "most commonly created by a technique in which high quality pot is blasted with butane that is then extracted, these *cannabis* concentrates approach 70 to 90 percent THC."[22]

Q: What is hash oil?

A: Hash oils are similar are another concentrate and they are typically very dark in color and very sticky. It's more

---

[22] "The Amateur's Guide to Dabs - Alexander Abad-Santos - The Atlantic Wire." Accessed September 14, 2013. http://www.theatlanticwire.com/national/2013/05/amateurs-guide-dabs/65266/.

difficult to work with oils than with waxes in terms of handling them because they are either thin like oil to thick and sticky and stringy. When I first started out I bought several types of oil. I assumed they were the same strength and quality as wax, but in another form. Oils are generally lower quality than budder, wax and shatter and they don't taste as good either. I also noticed that the vapor that I get from oil is much thinner and weaker than that of budder, wax or shatter.

Dispensaryweed.com explains, hash oil is usually "The result of a resin separation process that is sticky and black. It's usually indicative of very old or low quality source material, but it can also be the result of too much heat and a novice hash maker." He also goes on to explain that "if it's black at least you know it's been purged well, even if it is too well".[23]

Q: What is a pre-roll?

A: A pre-roll is a pre-rolled marijuana cigarette, also called a joint. Sometimes clubs will sell pre-rolls of the smaller (but just as potent) buds or even mixtures of all kinds. Typically you will find the mixed pre-rolls at a cheaper price. I've seen people buy the budget pre-rolls and take them home and empty the buds out and consume them in another way, just because it was cheaper that way.

---

[23] "Differences Between Wax and Budder - Concentrated Cannabis - WeedTRACKER." Accessed September 14, 2013. http://dispensaryweed.com/cannabis/topic/193441-differences-between-wax-and-budder/.

THE CALIFORNIA MEDICAL MARIJUANA PATIENTS BOOK

Q: Is it necessary to sterilize marijuana plant material and buds before use?

A: Patients who have compromised immune systems may be advised by their doctors to sterilize marijuana before using or consuming it. Aspergillus is a fungus sometimes found on marijuana and the spores from this fungus can cause serious lung infections in these patients.

These pathogen and fungus issues can occur when marijuana is dried improperly. It must be dried until the moisture content is between 10% and 15%. When it's too low your marijuana will be unusually brittle and will crumble easily. When it's too high, you risk fungal growth.

This is really important for any patient with a weak immune system. Other patients do not typically sterilize their marijuana.

Q: Do I need to sterilize concentrates?

A: Concentrates that have been extracted are already sterilized as part of the heating process that extracts and purges the concentrates.

Q: How do I sterilize marijuana?

A: If your marijuana has visible mold spores on it then pot is unusable and should be thrown away. Even if you sterilize the marijuana, it will still contain unknown fungal toxins created by the mold and these can make you extremely ill.

To sterilize marijuana, you simply place it on a cookie sheet in your oven (heated at 300F degrees) for five minutes. This

T. OLIVER

process will kill Aspergillus, if it's present.

THE CALIFORNIA MEDICAL MARIJUANA PATIENTS BOOK

CHAPTER EIGHT

Growing Q & A

Q: How many plants can I grow?

A: California State Senate Bill 420 allows patients with written recommendations to possess up to six (6) mature plants, twelve (12) immature plants, and (8) eight ounces of dried cannabis. Individual city and county governments may pass laws to increase the allowances but they may not pass laws that reduce these numbers.

Q: What's the local law regarding growing allowance in my area?

A: California NORML (http://bit.ly/197hhfC) keeps a regular list of the changing local growing allowances for each county

SafeAccessNow.com (http://bit.ly/197p7UC) also provides an excellent list of city and county laws that affect medical marijuana patients allowances

T. OLIVER

Q: Is there a limit on the size of the room where I will grow?

A: SB420 does not limit the size of a grow room. It simply states you are limited to six (6) mature plants or twelve (12) immature plants as well as 1/2 lb. (8 oz.) of processed plant material.

Some local laws do address growing space. These laws change so frequently that you should again check online sources. Some local city and county laws specify square footage for your grow space.

Be sure to check the sources above regarding local ordinances.

Q: Can I grow if I rent my home or apartment?

A: Unfortunately, landlords in California may exclude the use and/or cultivation of medical marijuana in their leases. It's advisable to keep your use or cultivation of your medicine as low key as possible.

I spoke to the owner of a very large property management company here in Santa Rosa, he said their company was Prop 215 friendly as long as the patients stayed within the state limits and that they didn't get any complaints.

When renting, it's a good idea to grow indoors, as outdoor plants seem to attract a lot of attention of neighbors and thieves. Even if a Prop 215 friendly rental, flaunting it can cause you problems if people complain or if a landlord decides they want you to move out.

Some Craigslist searches turned up rental and roommate ads that said 'Prop 215' or '215 friendly'. If it's important to you, try finding a landlord that is 215 friendly.

If for some reason you have problems with renting or your landlord you can contact a NORML attorney (http://bit.ly/1eCvh2v) in your area.

Q: Where can I get information on growing?

A: I'm not an expert on growing and this isn't a how to grow book but I can offer you a few really great online resources for learning how to grow marijuana.

- www.growweedeasy.com
  http://bit.ly/1fOfh0m

- www.howtogrowmarijuana.com
  http://bit.ly/1a0Vng8

- www.rollitup.org
  http://bit.ly/19VjZB6

- www.growingmarijuana.com
  http://bit.ly/1a0Vw3a

On top of these great resources you can also find lots of books on amazon that will help you start your home garden.

Q: I have children; can I still grow in my household?

A: Yes, you can still grow your own medicine legally. It's advisable that you're very careful to not let children get around your medication. You should grow your own medicine in an area that can be locked where children won't have access.

If you're sharing custody of your child with an ex, you should be aware that growing or using marijuana can possibly come up in court and may be used against you.

Q: Can I grow in my backyard?

A: Yes, you can grow outdoors on your property. You should be aware that if you grow outdoors and you're in an area where people can see it, someone might try to steal your crop or even complain about it. I've heard many stories of people growing in their yards and having no problems until it comes time to harvest and someone sweeps into their backyard and steals all of their mature plants. Be cautious about where you grow and don't tell everyone you know about your crop or it may not be your crop for long.

If you're in a neighborhood with homes that are close together you should also be aware that occasionally patients have had the police come and take their crops after receiving complaints from neighbors, even when they are within the legal limits.

For the most part, outdoor gardens are only recommended if you can do it discretely. Maybe you have an area in your yard that is private or you're lucky enough to have a large property, outdoor growing may be for you. If you do have property where you can grow then I can offer some tips for securing your garden.

TIPS! - OUTDOOR GARDEN SECURITY

- If your garden is in the woods or through a field, do

not leave trails to your garden. Cover up your tracks or use a different path to the garden each time.

- Don't bring people with you. The minute you start telling your friend, brother, cousin and they mention it to someone else; you've lost your crop and even possibly invited a robbery. My cousin told his brother, who shared it with a friend; their crop was stolen two days before they planned to harvest it.

- Don't attract attention to your grow site. Clean up your mess. Don't leave behind garbage. Don't use someone else's private property without permission.

- Avoid patterns in growing such as rows. These are easily picked out from above. Your garden will be less visible if it's random and amongst other plants and foliage. Don't plant out in the open; make sure there is some coverage but not so much that your plants won't get sunlight.

- Either purchase animal repellant or urine or you can urinate around your grow site to keep away the wild animals.

- Visit your garden in the early morning or at night. Avoid using flashlights at night.

- If it's in your backyard and you live in a neighborhood where your neighbors are close, you may have a hard time keeping your garden a secret and keeping people from stealing it from you. You are also more likely to have neighbors complaining. Think about this before choosing an outdoor garden.

T. OLIVER

TIPS! - INDOOR GARDEN SECURITY

- DO NOT TELL ANYONE about your garden. This is first and foremost. Most police involvement is due to a tip off. You tell your friend, who tells their brother, who tells a friend and now you have the potential for a robbery or dealing with the police.

- If you are buying a lot of equipment or materials do not unload it all in broad daylight. Hauling in a bunch of lights and 20 bags of soil is going to look suspicious. Wait until later in the evening to unload the car.

- Be careful of light leaks. Use heavy drapery or even black out shades. Check for leaks of the grow lights from the outdoors.

- Keep your indoor grow room in a locked area. If a guest accidentally opens the door, you grow room is no longer a secret. This also a very important so that you keep children out of your grow room.

- Control the smell. You can vent the room with filters and other methods. If your marijuana is super smelly you should research online how to vent the room properly.

Q: What are the benefits of growing my own medical marijuana?

A: There are many benefits, all of which I am sure I won't cover here but here's the basics. You control your medicine and you know exactly what was in that medicine. You can grow organic medicine. It's more economical to grow your own cannabis, as there is quite a markup at the dispensaries. Growing your own quality medicine will take some startup costs in equipment but you will quickly make back the cost of that equipment with one or two good harvests. You may have a learning curve to deal with when growing, so keep that in mind.

Q: What are some potential downsides of growing my own medicine?

A: You have to have the space and equipment to grow. You either need some level of automation or you will need to be dedicated to taking care of your plants regularly. Growing requires a little bit of a green thumb, so there can be a learning curve in producing a really nice crop. I personally really enjoy having several different strains of meds for different uses and only growing my meds would limit to me to many fewer strains. Though I have grown in the past; I currently am strictly a dispensary/cooperative/delivery customer at the moment because I do not have a good grow space.

Q: Can I give away marijuana I have grown if I have extra?

A: Legally, you should not have extra as the law states you can grow only as much as you need for your condition. This is another grey area. You could potentially get into legal trouble if for some reason you gave it away and the person then had a run in with law enforcement; should they chose to name you as the grower you may have legal trouble. Anyone who receives medical marijuana must have a valid recommendation. Many people grow and give away extra to friends and family but you should be aware that this is not legal and this is generally done discretely.

Q: Can I sell my extra medicine to other patients or collectives?

A: You cannot really 'sell' your extra medication. The law permits you to grow only what you need. You can join collectives and possibly grow for that collective. This allows you to recoup your costs for the production of the marijuana through the 'donations' that the other members will give for the medication. You will likely need to develop a relationship with a particular collective before you can grow for them. Some collectives are choosier than others; some will buy anything that looks halfway decent.

Q: What is a collective cultivation authorization?

A: Some collectives will provide members who grow with a collective cultivation authorization or a vendor authorization document. Other collectives will require you to provide the document for them to sign. The document will prove that you are a member of the collective and you are growing for the collective and the other members. Post this on your grow room along with a copy of your recommendation.

Q: Can I get a grower's license so I can grow more?

A: There is no such thing as a grower's license. There is no state license for growing. Doctor's cannot legally issue a license for growing marijuana. Any doctor or office offering such a license, is shady, and putting you at great legal risk. These shady doctors usually offer these 'licenses' for a much

THE CALIFORNIA MEDICAL MARIJUANA PATIENTS BOOK

higher fee, some fees as high as $250.

Because the law allows a patient to grow as much medicine as necessary for their condition these doctors may write a recommendation saying they think that patient needs to grow 50 plants. The problem with this situation is that when and if you ever have an issue with law enforcement you will have to prove that you actually needed 50 plants for your condition. The doctor who wrote it will likely not come to your defense. You will need to hire a lawyer and will likely have to argue that you were cultivating marijuana for a collective as a defense.

Q: How much does a grow area setup cost to start?

A: Setting up your own grow room can run from $100 in basic used equipment for a small setup up in to the thousands for the ultimate grow room. More money will buy you better quality equipment as well as more automation.

You can grow great medicine on a $500 setup or you can spend more and get an amazing setup that is more automated. I deluxe, large, grow room can cost as much as $10,000, though at this amount you are likely growing much more than you can consume.

My suggestion is that you do some research on growing and setups. Go talk to your local growing supply shop. Look on craigslist for people selling their used equipment. You'll pay a fraction of the original cost.

T. OLIVER

Q: Do I just buy seeds and start growing?

A: Luckily in California, we have choices. There are not many states where you can walk into a store and walk out with clones of your favorite strain.

Some people opt for buying clones from the various clubs and growers around the state. Clones are cuttings from a mother plant, so it's genetically the same as the mother plant. Clones will shorten your growing cycle by approximately one month. If you buy clones then you should be careful who and where you obtain these clones. If the mother plant had problems then you will inherit those problems. You will want to ask if the club sells marijuana grown from the same clones or if it's from another source.

Seeds can be obtained from reputable seed banks. You can even buy feminized seeds from seed banks so that you can almost guarantee that all your plants will be female. If you use non-feminized seeds then at least half of your plants will be male, and therefore, useless to you. Seeds will give you the best chance of starting out without pests or disease.

THE CALIFORNIA MEDICAL MARIJUANA PATIENTS BOOK

ABOUT THE AUTHOR

My name is T. Oliver, but my friends call me Ollie. I live in beautiful Sonoma County, about 45 minutes north of the Golden Gate Bridge in San Francisco. I enjoy reading, graphic design, spending time with family and friends and just about anything technology related.

My personal journey with chronic illness and pain and navigating our medical system is how I started using medical marijuana and it's how this book was born.

Medical marijuana has changed my life, it's saved me in a way. I have a fairly severe case of Ulcerative Colitis and spent over a year being horribly ill and depressed (for the first time in my life) because of the illness. I never thought I could really be depressed but once I found myself helplessly ill to the point of not being able to enjoy life, I was consumed with depression and sickness.

When I am sick, my body hurts all over and I'm nauseous constantly. During these times, eating makes me feel sick and an empty stomach guarantees I will feel even more nauseous. I tried all the medications the doctors could prescribe and even ended up in the emergency room a few times for pain management during flare ups of my disease.

Did I mention that I hate the way pain killers make me feel and I'm terrified of addiction? The pain killers didn't work very well and the side effects I experienced as a result of taking pain killers weren't fun; constipation, itching, and extreme irritability. Even when I took the pain killers, I was still left with the nausea and the pills often made the nausea even worse.

T. OLIVER

Never mind that these controlled substances had a long scary list of side effects and they were also terribly addictive.

For over a year I tried to figure out how I could live with this pain and nausea and still work and have a life that I could enjoy with my family. After many months of trying out all the traditional pharmaceuticals and having no success I began my research to get a valid recommendation and an ID card.

Marijuana helps me manage my nausea and pain and I live a full life. It's done for me what no one in traditional medicine could. Not only does it helps me cope with my symptoms on a daily basis but I believe it has actually helped me manage my disease and help to keep it under control. I had three painful flare ups in my first year; one that lasted several months. I've not had one full flare up of my disease since I began using medical marijuana in the last four years.

It's been my miracle drug. I hope it's yours too.

T. Oliver

P.S.

If you believe the book is worth sharing, and you think you have friends and family that would like it, would you take a moment to let your friends know about it by leaving a review on Amazon or Goodreads? If it turns out to make a difference in their lives, they'll forever be grateful to you. As I will.

www.ingramcontent.com/pod-product-compliance
Lightning Source LLC
Chambersburg PA
CBHW051804170526
45167CB00005B/1881